Aromatherapy
for Beginners

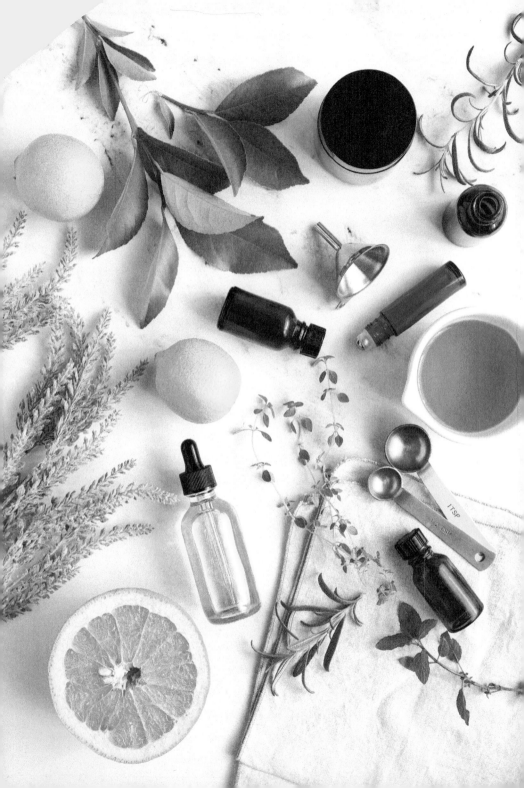

Aromatherapy *for* Beginners

THE COMPLETE GUIDE TO
Getting Started with Essential Oils

Anne Kennedy

PHOTOGRAPHY BY HÉLÈNE DUJARDIN

ALTHEA
PRESS

For Mary, Ellie, Dominic, Maggie, Vincent, Bernadette, Monica, Regina, Joe, and Claire: You, my brothers and sisters, are the brightest flowers in the garden of life.

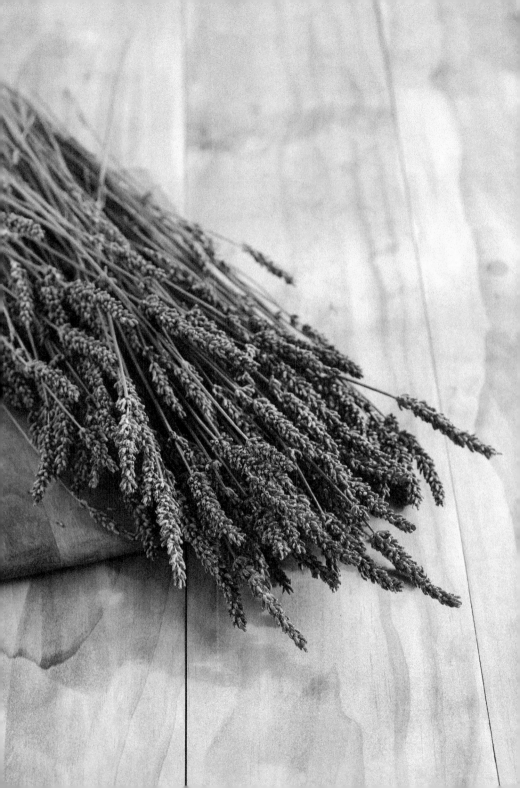

Contents

PART TWO Remedies, Recipes, & Applications

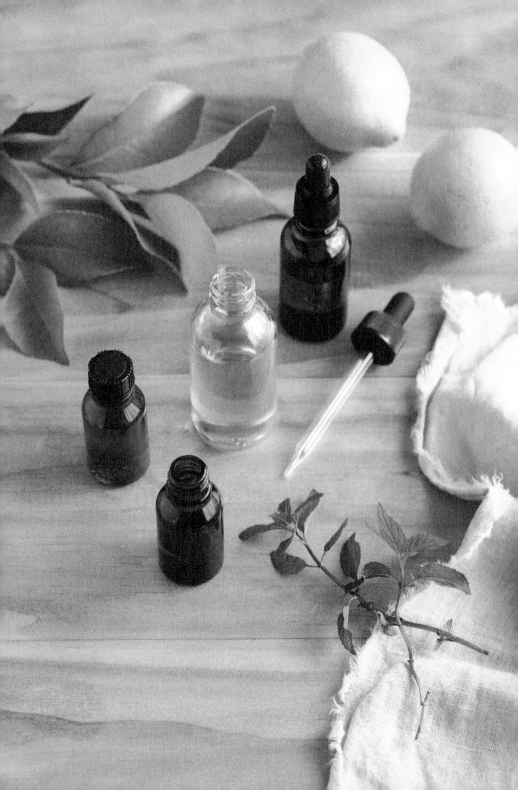

Introduction

Several years ago, a stressful life change turned my world upside-down. It was then that a good friend introduced me to my first essential oil: lavender. Its ability to help me de-stress was nothing short of incredible, and I loved the way it helped me drop off to sleep even when I was feeling anxious and overwrought.

I tried peppermint oil next. I caught a nasty stomach bug and the same friend encouraged me to try it for nausea. I was skeptical, even though I was no stranger to herbal and homeopathic remedies. Despite my misgivings, I was desperate enough to put a few drops of peppermint essential oil on the soles of my feet. The relief was almost immediate, leaving me both grateful and intrigued—I was hooked! How could something so simple (and weird?) work so well?

Soon, I was experimenting with aromatherapy and digging deep into books about it. I learned to create some of my own blends, making some "interesting" mistakes along the way. Luckily, essential oils are forgiving. An overpowering blend is easily toned down with the addition of more carrier oil, and an unappealing mixture can be used in a nontoxic household cleanser if adding other oils fails to redeem it.

My introduction to essential oils happened before aromatherapy enjoyed the surge in popularity that has brought it into common use today. There were a few good companies offering quality essential oils at the time, but availability was limited, and prices were higher.

These days, there are many more essential oils and blends to choose from, and they are easier to find. It's great to have so many options, but there is also lots of marketing hype surrounding certain essential oils and brands. This can create some confusion for beginners. Do I have the right oils? Do I have the best brand? Am I going to be harmed because I don't have essential oils from a company that claims its products are superior to others?

Relax! You don't need to buy every essential oil to reap the benefits of aromatherapy. It's nice to have an extensive collection, but you don't need everything all at once.

Many people work with a small number of favorites; you can meet most of your everyday needs with a small number of versatile essential oils. Whether you've already purchased a starter kit that contains popular basics, such as lavender, peppermint, eucalyptus, and tea tree, or are still deciding which essential oils to begin with, it's easy to put them to use with this book as your guide.

These pages offer an introduction to the world of aromatherapy in a factual, friendly way, providing complete profiles of 15 top essential oils—nine "must haves" (clove, eucalyptus, geranium, lavender, lemon, lemongrass, peppermint, rosemary, and tea tree) and six "great to haves" (clary sage, frankincense, grapefruit, patchouli, Roman chamomile, and thyme), which includes those found in most starter kits. While anyone can buy essential oils and start diffusing them right away, this approach is different:

- You'll begin by learning five easy steps to exploring aromatherapy safely.

- You will build a strong foundation of knowledge, and gain the confidence to incorporate this wonderful practice into your everyday life.

This book contains more than 150 useful recipes and applications to help you use these 15 essential oils to their fullest potential. And, it's easy to find exactly what you want at a glance, using a special label for recipes that use the nine "must-have" oils. Many are meant to complement Western medicine and promote natural wellness. Others are wonderful alternatives to toxic or expensive commercial products for body and home.

I use essential oils on a daily basis, from addressing minor health issues, to creating my own aromatherapy self-care and household products. It is my hope you will find just as much pleasure in these beautiful, natural oils as I do.

Your knowledge of essential oils will grow and expand over time—no need to be in a hurry. Savor the process and discover the many ways in which aromatherapy can enhance your life. Soon, you'll be enjoying them to their fragrant fullest.

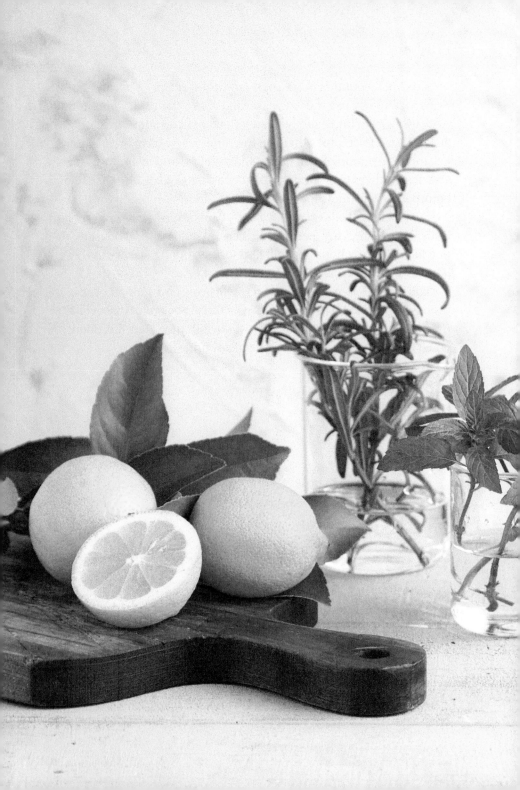

PART ONE

The Power of Aromatherapy

You're about to embark on an exploration of aromatherapy. The first part of this book is designed to help you become comfortable with and knowledgeable of some basic concepts, and learn common terminology. How do essential oils work? What are the most popular—and safest—ways to use these oils to enhance your daily life? What should you look for, and what's best to avoid? These are just a few of the questions answered here.

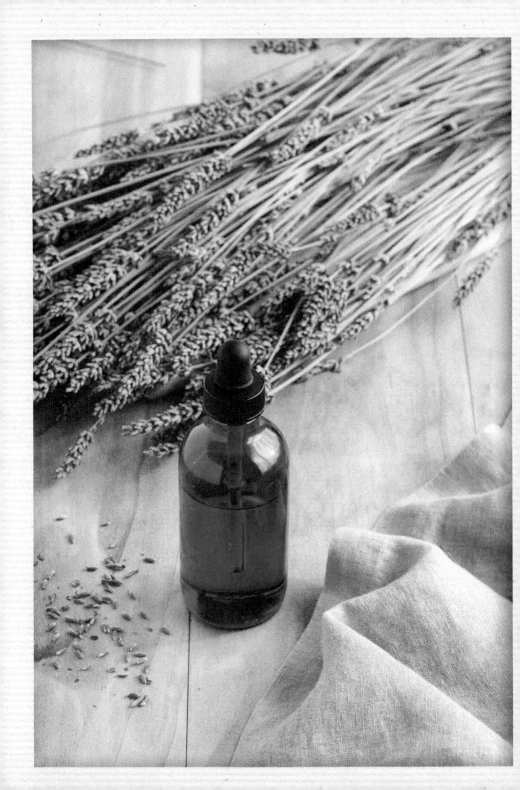

Aromatherapy for Health and Well-Being

You've heard the term before and you may already know its definition: *Aromatherapy* is a method of using essential oils to improve quality of life. The "aroma" part of the word tells you how this therapeutic practice works: When an essential oil's fragrance reaches your nose, you also inhale microscopic particles of the oil itself. These tiny droplets contain potent chemical components that can relieve common cold symptoms, ease tension, and more. Blended and applied topically, these same constituents can perform a variety of functions: some provide natural pain relief, others help minor wounds heal faster, and still others discourage bugs from biting.

There are hundreds of essential oils and premade blends on the market, and this may make you think you need an extensive collection to enjoy aromatherapy's benefits. The good news is, it takes very few essential oils to start. In fact, you can begin experimenting with just one oil that appeals to you and build your personal apothecary as your comfort level increases. Choose a few of the most versatile, must-have oils, and you'll be well on your way to enjoying a variety of aromatherapy's most appealing benefits.

The Science of Essential Oils

People have been using essential oils for centuries—not just for their pleasant aromas, but to treat a wide array of ailments. For much of this time, physicians saw that certain oils had specific effects, but they didn't know how or why these treatments worked so well.

Science is finally beginning to show us how essential oils interact with organisms, including viruses and bacteria. Thanks to a growing body of research, including some remarkable clinical studies, we now know far more about the ways in which aromatherapy works. This chapter provides a brief overview of the science of essential oils.

Powerful Plant Extracts

When you read an essential oil's label or description, you may see notes about the production method used to extract it from the source plant. This is by no means an exhaustive discussion of extraction methods; instead, it's a quick introduction to some of the most common.

DISTILLATION

This is among the oldest of all extraction methods, yet it remains popular. Aromatic plant matter, such as lavender flowers or rosemary leaves, is packed into a sealed chamber. Steam from a nearby pressure system is introduced, gently breaking down the plant matter and releasing volatile oils. The now-fragrant steam is carried into a condenser, where the steam and essential oils are cooled. The resulting liquid flows into a separate chamber, where the essential oil naturally separates from the water and is siphoned off. The leftover water, called hydrosol, retains a strong fragrance and, thus, carries some of the essential oil's benefits. It often makes its way into perfumes, lotions, and other personal care products.

Purity

There's a lot of discussion about this topic out there, including arguments about which companies offer the highest quality oils, etc. Certain extraction methods work better for some plants than others—for example, citrus oils don't withstand heat well, and there are questions about plant quality from one harvest to the next. Some even argue that mixing plants from different batches or crops results in an inferior finished product.

I personally check to ensure the essential oil in question is the only ingredient listed on the bottle, unless I'm picking up a prediluted oil, such as rose or jasmine, in which case the additional ingredient is a carrier oil such as sweet almond. Also, I try to ensure purity by purchasing my essential oils from reputable companies. My nose— and the way I feel when I smell the essential oils—tell me I've made a good choice.

COLD PRESSING

Also known as expression, cold pressing is the most common method of obtaining citrus oils. In cold pressing, the citrus rinds are macerated while spinning in a chamber, which breaks the tiny, oil-filled sacs on the fruit's skin. The resulting fluid is spun rapidly to create centrifugal force, separating the essential oil from the liquid.

HYPERCRITICAL CO_2 EXTRACTION

Essential oils labeled as CO_2 extracts are produced using this highly technical process in which plant matter is blended with pressurized, liquefied carbon dioxide. The process is similar to distilling, however no water remains in the collection chamber.

Instead, the CO_2 returns to its gaseous form when pressure is released, and only the essential oil remains. The finished product is usually more expensive than the same essential oil produced from traditional distillation.

How Essential Oils Work

While some manufacturers market essential oils for internal use, *it's best to take a very cautious approach to assure your safety and ensure anything you take internally is labeled for dietary use.* This book does not discourage internal use, but it focuses on traditional aromatherapy methods that rely on inhalation and topical use, which allow beneficial molecules to enter the body and provide beneficial effects.

When inhaled: The fragrance from an essential oil carries molecules into the nose, where they stimulate smell receptors and interact with the body's nervous and limbic systems. The limbic system is a deep, primal portion of the brain responsible for controlling emotion.

At the same time, essential oil particles are delivered to the lungs with each breath. There, they enter the bloodstream and are carried throughout the entire body, where they act directly on the brain and other organs. A 2015 study published in the *Journal of Alternative and Complementary Medicine* showed impressive results. One group of subjects applied inhalation patches containing lavender essential oil to their chests each night. A second control group wore blank patches. The group using lavender enjoyed better sleep.

When applied topically: While the aroma enters your lungs and nostrils, even more molecules are absorbed into your skin. This often provides an immediate benefit: stopping the itch from a mosquito bite, soothing the pain from a sunburn, or taking some of the sting out of a minor wound.

Just one essential oil can provide a variety of benefits. Clove, for example, is capable of repelling mosquitoes and numbing pain. At the same time, it is a powerful antifungal agent, as shown in a 2009 study published in the *Journal of Medical Microbiology*. It has the ability to destroy *Candida albicans*—the fungus that causes yeast infections—and other fungi, including some strains that resist the antifungal drug fluconazole backs up its traditional use as a remedy for common fungal infections such as athlete's foot and jock itch.

The Benefits of Using Essential Oils

Aromatherapy can provide natural, nonpharmaceutical relief for a variety of symptoms and can replace some over-the-counter medications. For example, peppermint oil can help soothe indigestion, ease cold symptoms, and stop headaches. If you need a quick energy boost or a way to wind down, aromatherapy can help. Just add a few drops of rosemary to your shower for an energizing morning boost, or diffuse frankincense to ground yourself after a hectic rush-hour commute.

With a few deodorizing and germ-killing essential oils, you can keep your home fresh and clean. By mixing a little bit of clove, lemon, or tea tree essential oil with simple, inexpensive ingredients such as baking soda or rubbing alcohol, you can create homemade cleansers that replace a cupboard full of toxic concoctions with scary warning labels. Lavender is a fantastic example of a versatile essential oil: It can be diffused to freshen a room, provide a relaxing atmosphere, applied topically to treat minor injuries and irritations, and mixed into cleansers for your home. You can even use it to help keep fleas from pestering your pets.

With essential oils, a little goes a long way. And since most recipes call for just a few drops, when you choose aromatherapy and use your essential oils frequently, you'll save money, especially if you're already paying top dollar for natural brands. The recipes in

Glossary of Aromatherapy Terms

These common terms describing properties of essential oils will help you decide which essential oil provides the benefits you're looking for.

ABSOLUTE: alcohol-based essential oil extract with 5 to 10 parts per million of solvent residue remaining from the extraction process

ADULTERATED: oil containing anything but pure, 100-percent essential oil

ANESTHETIC: relives pain or offers a numbing effect

ANTIBIOTIC: destroys bacteria or prevents its growth

ANTI-INFLAMMATORY: prevents or reduces inflammation

ANTISPASMODIC: helps prevent cramping and/or muscle spasms

ANTIVIRAL: fights viral infections

APERITIF: a substance that stimulates appetite

ASTRINGENT: encourages tissues to tighten

BULKING: using plants from the same species but from different harvests to reduce the cost of a specific oil

CARMINATIVE: facilitates healthy digestion and prevents gas formation in the digestive tract

CEPHALIC: a substance that stimulates the mind

CHOLAGOGUE: promotes the release of bile encouraging better digestion

CICATRIZANT: promotes healing and the formation of healthy scar tissue

CORDIAL: a substance that provides a feeling of invigoration

CYTOPHYLACTIC: stimulates cellular growth or regeneration

EMMENAGOGUE: stimulates or promotes menstruation

EMOLLIENT: softens skin

EUPHORIC: promotes feelings of happiness

EXPECTORANT: encourages the elimination of mucus

FEBRIFUGE: fever reducer

HEPATIC: a substance that stimulates the liver

NERVINE: a substance that relaxes the nervous system

RUBEFACIENT: increases circulation and reddens the skin

SUDORIFIC: a substance that promotes perspiration

TONIC: a substance that restores or strengthens energy

VASOCONSTRICTOR: promotes blood vessel contraction

VERMIFUGE: purges intestinal parasites

VULNERARY: encourages wound healing

this book are designed to help you take advantage of all these benefits, whether you choose just a few oils or treat yourself to a robust starter kit.

Safety Precautions and Best Practices

Why worry about safety? Aren't essential oils just plant extracts? While it's true that essential oils are natural, it's also true they are highly concentrated—and can come from some of the most potent plants on the planet. There is no reason to fear any of the essential oils in this book as long as you use them appropriately. Essential oil safety isn't complicated, so by taking just a few simple precautions, you can enjoy their many benefits without worry or overexposure.

Less is Truly More

It takes an enormous amount of plant matter to make just one drop of essential oil. For example, it takes about 60 roses to make a single drop of pure rose essential oil—no wonder it's expensive! Cost isn't the only reason to approach essential oil use with a judicious hand; every drop of essential oil contains the concentrated chemical components from all the plants that went into it, so there is a risk of overuse. Using too much essential oil can cause adverse effects, just like using too much medicine.

Even though these are natural remedies and are generally safe—improper or excessive use can be dangerous. It's important to approach aromatherapy mindfully and respect these natural medicines the same way you respect prescription and drugstore remedies. By using only the amount required, you'll receive the benefits you need, you'll save money, and you won't risk injury, irritation, or illness.

Safety Tips

- Always conduct a patch test before trying a new oil. Moisten a cotton ball with 3 to 4 drops of carrier oil (see page 25), add 1 drop of essential oil to the cotton ball, and dab the cotton ball on the inner fold of an elbow. Cover the spot with a bandage and check for irritation 24 hours later.

- Keep essential oils out of reach of children and pets. Warn older children about the dangers of overexposure.

- Infants, toddlers, and children under age 12 are often highly sensitive to essential oils. Elderly people and those with compromised immune systems may be very sensitive, too. Be cautious about overexposure and use extra care with patch tests.

- If you're allergic to certain plants or plant families, avoid all essential oils that come from those plants.

- Some essential oils cause photosensitization, meaning they can increase your risk of sunburn. If you use an essential oil with a photosensitization warning, avoid sun exposure and tanning beds for 6 to 24 hours after application, depending on the individual essential oil and the warning that accompanies it.

- Some essential oils may be used undiluted on skin. If you have sensitive skin, you may want to dilute each drop of essential oil with a drop of carrier oil, even if that essential oil is generally safe to use undiluted.

- A few essential oils are safe for use during pregnancy and breastfeeding, but most should be avoided—even if the risks are minor or aren't well-documented.

- Many essential oils can irritate or injure eyes and mucous membranes, so use them carefully. If accidental contact occurs, flush the area thoroughly with water.

- Essential oils are flammable. Keep them away from open flames and ignition sources.

Best Practices

- Know your essential oils. Research them before you purchase to help you avoid unwanted side effects and ensure you're able to use each oil for a variety of purposes.

- Think about your needs, and then decide which oils will meet them. Assure their safety by checking for contraindications, and check with your doctor if you take any prescription medicines. For example, grapefruit essential oil acts much like grapefruit, interacting with certain medications.

- It's a good idea to switch essential oils every now and then. It's possible to build a tolerance to their effects, and using a strong remedy in the same area for several days or weeks can cause skin irritation. Pay close attention to how your oils affect your body. If, for example, you diffuse lavender at bedtime but you're still feeling wakeful, try another relaxing oil instead, such as clary sage.

Using Starter Essential Oils as Substitutes

Dig deeper into the world of aromatherapy and you'll notice that many essential oils offer similar benefits to one another, and others have similar scents. In many cases, it's possible to use one essential oil in place of another—which is especially nice when a recipe calls for something expensive and you'd rather save your money.

Listed here are 25 of the world's most expensive essential oils, plus some possible substitutions you can try.

You'll notice some of these costly oils have scents that can't be recreated by substituting another oil; these fragrances are uniquely complex. Many of the most expensive oils are primarily used in perfumery, even though they often come with psychotherapeutic effects. Additional discussion about essential oil substitutions appears in chapter 2.

Agarwood

SCENT: No substitute
ACTION: Try frankincense for a similarly uplifting experience.

Angelica

SCENT: Try a drop of clary sage, which has a similar green, woody aroma.
ACTION: Try rosemary, or lavender for a similar grounding, detoxifying effect. Try a drop of clary sage for similar relief from menstrual and menopausal symptoms.

Calendula CO$_2$

SCENT: No substitute
ACTION: Try lavender or frankincense for a similar soothing, healing effect. Preblended calendula oil is another option.

Carnation

SCENT: No substitute
ACTION: Try clary sage for a similar aphrodisiac effect.

German (Blue) Chamomile

SCENT: Roman chamomile shares a similar scent profile; the two are not identical but can easily stand in for each other.
ACTION: Try clove for a similar pain relief effect. Try Roman chamomile for a similar relaxing effect.

Helichrysum

SCENT: Try blending a drop of lavender with a drop of clary sage for a similar fresh, herbaceous scent.
ACTION: Try lavender, frankincense, or patchouli for a similar healing effect.

Hops

SCENT: No substitute
ACTION: Try lavender, Roman chamomile, or clary sage for a similar sedative effect.

Hyssop

SCENT: Try blending a drop of clary sage and a drop of peppermint or rosemary to replicate hyssop's very light, fresh, herbal fragrance.
ACTION: Try lavender, patchouli, or tea tree for a similar antiviral effect.

Jasmine

SCENT: No substitute
ACTION: Try lavender or geranium for a similar skin-soothing effect. Try clary sage for similar relief from menstrual and menopausal symptoms.

Lotus

SCENT: No substitute
ACTION: Try patchouli or frankincense for a similar meditative experience.

Melissa

SCENT: Try blending a drop of peppermint or clary sage with 2 drops of lemon for a similar fresh, lemony fragrance.
ACTION: Try clary sage or lavender for a similar relaxing effect. Try rosemary for similar relief from respiratory discomfort.

Myrrh

SCENT: Try frankincense for a fragrance that shares a similar richness and warmth.
ACTION: Try frankincense, lavender, or geranium for similar skin-healing effects.

Neroli

SCENT: No substitute
ACTION: Try lavender, clary sage, or patchouli for similar relief from stress and anxiety.

Oakmoss

SCENT: No substitute
ACTION: Try peppermint or rosemary for similar relief from congestion.

Palo Santo

SCENT: Try frankincense; the two are close relatives and their scents share some similar qualities.
ACTION: Try frankincense for similar anti-inflammatory and pain-relieving effects.

(CONTINUED ON NEXT PAGE)

Rose

SCENT: No substitute, but preblended rose oil is an inexpensive option worth exploring.
ACTION: Try geranium for similar skin-soothing effects.

Sandalwood

SCENT: No substitute
ACTION: Try frankincense for similar skin-soothing effects.

Spikenard

SCENT: Try clary sage as a stand-in for spikenard's strong, earthy fragrance.
ACTION: Try clary sage for similar relief from menstrual symptoms. Use lavender, clary sage, or patchouli for similar relief from stress and anxiety.

St. John's Wort

SCENT: Try diluting 1 drop of clary sage with 5 or 6 drops of carrier oil for a similarly light, herbal fragrance.
ACTION: Try geranium or Roman chamomile for similar skin-soothing effects. Try rosemary for increasing mental clarity in a similar, but less pronounced, way.

Vanilla CO₂

SCENT: No substitute
ACTION: Try frankincense, Roman chamomile, or lavender for a similar relaxing effect.

Vetiver

SCENT: No substitute
ACTION: Try lavender or clary sage for a similar soothing, relaxing effect. Topically, try tea tree or lavender for minor cuts and scrapes.

Violet Leaf

SCENT: No substitute
ACTION: Try Roman chamomile or lavender for a similar relaxing effect. Topically, try geranium or lavender for soothing inflamed skin.

Vitex Berry

SCENT: Try blending 1 drop of lavender or geranium with 2 or 3 drops of clary sage for a somewhat similar herbal, earthy, slightly floral fragrance.
ACTION: Try clary sage for similar relief from menstrual and menopausal symptoms.

Ylang-Ylang

SCENT: No substitute
ACTION: Try clary sage or lavender for similar relief from insomnia. Clary sage also offers similar relief from menstrual and menopausal symptoms.

Yuzu

SCENT: Try grapefruit, lemon, or a combination of the two.
ACTION: Try grapefruit or lemon for a similarly uplifting sensation. Grapefruit and lemon readily stand in for other applications, such as increasing focus, reducing stress, and easing cold symptoms.

Your Starter Kit Essential Oil All-Stars

There are countless essential oils available, so how did just a handful make it onto this list? The criteria were simple. The 15 oils at the heart of this book were selected because they are versatile, affordable, and easy to find. Many come in starter kits from top essential oil companies, and all are fantastic for blending with a few others on the list.

Nine Must-Have Essential Oils

Clove   Lemongrass
Eucalyptus   Peppermint
Geranium   Rosemary
Lavender   Tea tree
Lemon

Six Great-to-Have Essential Oils

Clary sage   Patchouli
Frankincense   Roman chamomile
Grapefruit   Thyme

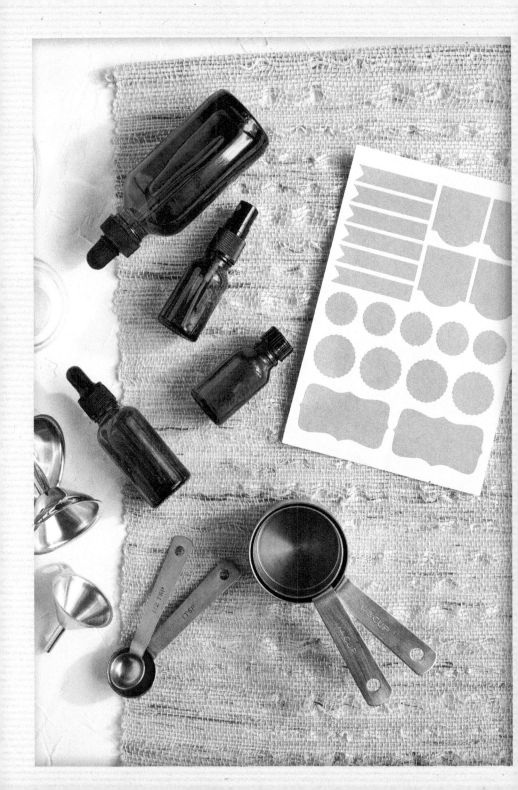

Working with Essential Oils

There are so many wonderful ways to put your essential oils to work in your life. They lend themselves to a wide range of uses—from freshening the air, revitalizing foot soaks, improving oral hygiene, soothing sore muscles, promoting clearer thinking, to relieving a wide variety of mild health complaints. You'll love the personalized blends you can create for use in your own bath and body care products, and you can use your oils to create thoughtful, yet inexpensive gifts for others. The sky is the limit!

Shopping for Essential Oils

When you begin shopping for essential oils—especially online—you'll notice there are many brands available, and each brand does its best to outshine its competitors. Take marketing claims with a grain of salt; it's very easy to find high-quality essential oils online, in stores, and from private distributors. Instead of focusing on buzzwords, it's most important to check that what's in the bottle is a *pure, natural essential oil.*

What to Look For

There are a few ways to check that an essential oil is of good quality. First, research the company that produces it and see what consumers have to say. It's normal to have a range of feedback; if the overall response is positive, you're likely to join the rest of the company's satisfied customers.

If you're purchasing a bottle of essential oil off the shelf, look for some key labeling components:

- Common name
- Latin name (genus and species, usually located beneath common name or under ingredients)
- Plant parts used, i.e., flowers or leaves
- Country of origin

Some companies include additional components on their labels:

- Extraction type
- Growing method
- Specific gas chromatography/mass spectrometry (GC/MS) data

Sometimes very expensive essential oils, such as rose and jasmine, are offered for sale prediluted in carrier oil. A percentage of oil might or might not be listed, but the seller will be very clear about what's in the bottle. Feel free to try these if you want to stretch your wings and experience some lovely, luxurious florals that might otherwise be outside your budget. If you are happy with other products from the same company, you'll likely enjoy using these.

Marketing Claims

Essential oil companies are understandably proud of their products. As part of the marketing process, companies often create terminology to convince potential customers that their products are superior to others. That's a normal part of doing business—and as a well-informed consumer, understanding marketing terminology helps you make the best choice.

100% Pure: People want to know they are purchasing unadulterated essential oils. This is one of the statements you'll find on some essential oils as a reassurance.

Aromatherapy Grade or Therapeutic Grade: There is no official grading system or oversight process for the production of essential oils; instead, companies set their own standards for quality.

Certified: Just as there is no official grading process, there is no official certification process for essential oils. Companies may have proprietary processes, but these are internal and have no bearing on the comparable quality of essential oils produced by other companies.

Popular Essential Oil Brands

This alphabetical list of some of the most popular essential oil brands is by no means exhaustive. The brands can serve as a starting point for your shopping research.

Aura Cacia

PROS: Wide selection of single and blended essential oils. Relatively low prices. Often carried by local venues.

CONS: Fewer options than some other brands.

doTERRA

PROS: Extensive catalogue of single and blended essential oils. Interactive customer service experience. Wholesale pricing available with membership.

CONS: Among the more expensive brands.

Edens Garden

PROS: Extensive catalogue of single and blended essential oils. Robust returns program. Low-cost samples are available. The company carries a variety of special blends for children.

CONS: Among the more expensive brands. Only available online.

Mountain Rose Herbs

PROS: Wide selection of single essential oils. Company has a good selection of bottles, tools, and ingredients.

CONS: No blends available. Only available online.

Nature's Bounty Earthly Elements

PROS: Low-cost, basic essential oils and blends. Often carried by local venues.

CONS: Fewer options than some other brands.

NOW Essential Oils

PROS: Good selection of the most popular essential oils. Relatively low prices. Often carried by local venues.

CONS: Fewer options than some other brands.

Plant Guru

PROS: Extensive selection of single and blended essential oils. Several value packs and starter kits. Lower prices than many other companies.

CONS: Only available online.

Rocky Mountain Oils

PROS: Extensive catalogue of single and blended essential oils. Robust customer satisfaction policy.

CONS: Among the more expensive brands.

Starwest Botanicals

PROS: Good selection of single and blended essential oils. Competitively priced. A good selection of bottles, tools, and ingredients.

CONS: Most products are only available online.

Young Living

PROS: Extensive catalogue of single and blended essential oils. Interactive customer service experience.

CONS: Among the more expensive brands.

What to Avoid

Most vendors offer essential oils in bottles made of dark-colored glass or lined aluminum that protects the oil from the oxidizing effect of light. Avoid essential oils packaged in clear glass containers, as well as plastic containers, even if those containers are dark-colored. One exception is bulk purchasing; if you are making lots of personal care products, you may find some reputable companies ship large quantities of essential oils in protective, BPA-free plastic bottles with instructions to transfer the essential oil to dark-colored glass containers as soon as possible. Skip essential oils packaged in bottles that come with rubber droppers on their lids. These look convenient, but will break down and cause contamination over time.

Be wary of essential oils that seem too cheap. A bargain is appealing, but might be low quality. Spend time researching prices, and you'll notice that some common oils, such as peppermint, lemon, and lavender, are fairly inexpensive as a rule, while others, such as patchouli and frankincense, cost a bit more. Look for a brand that offers products at a wide range of prices. Be suspicious if something like ylang-ylang (normally a pricy essential oil) costs the same as an inexpensive one like clove.

Be on the lookout for anything that simply sounds too good to be true. Always do your research before purchasing the product in question, and trust your intuition.

Look out for items labeled as *identical oil*, *perfume oil*, or *fragrance oil*. These are usually a combination of essential oil, carrier oil, and chemicals, usually offered for craft use. They are nice for making candles, but most aren't suitable for aromatherapy use.

Tools, Equipment, and Carrier Oils

You can create many of the recipes in this book with basic kitchen tools such as mixing bowls, measuring spoons, and measuring cups (metal or glass is preferred). Some do call for special containers, such as glass sugar shakers, which are inexpensive when purchased at large home goods retailers and online. What else might you need? The list of essentials is surprisingly short.

Essential Tools and Supplies

If you cook or bake, you may already have some of the tools and supplies needed for basic aromatherapy recipes. If you enjoy making your own bath and body products, you may want to invest in some separate tools at a later time; for now, you can let your existing items pull double duty. Most tools needed are metal or glass; this is because essential oils can melt plastic and, even if you can't see it happening, most plastics degrade with long-term contact with essential oils. There are a few exceptions, including bottles, lip balm tubes, and jars sold by essential oil companies.

Dark-colored glass bottles: These are ideal for storing your blends, smelling salts, and more. You can use clear bottles and jars, if needed and paint the outsides, cover them with athletic socks, or store them in a dark place to keep light out so your recipes last longer.

Diffuser: If you want to scent your home naturally and enjoy the many psychotherapeutic benefits of aromatherapy, invest in at least one diffuser. There are a variety of sizes, colors, and styles available.

Funnels: From tiny, purpose-built funnels that fit essential oil bottles to large, wide-mouth funnels that fit quart jars, these keep spills to a minimum when transferring finished products into storage containers.

Glass or metal mixing bowls: It's best to have a variety of sizes for holding ingredients and blending recipes.

Measuring cups and spoons: Glass or metal measuring cups and spoons are necessary for many recipes. Just one liquid measuring cup marked in ounce and cup increments can perform many functions.

Spray bottles: Small, glass bottles are best for aromatherapy products, but standard plastic spray bottles are fine for household cleaners.

Stainless steel pans: These are good for warming carrier oils and very carefully melting waxes.

Tape or labels: You'll want to carefully mark all of your blends and recipes with permanent marker. Printable labels are nice to have, especially if you enjoy treating others to homemade aromatherapy blends.

Whisks and metal spoons: These are great for blending recipes, but avoid wood because it absorbs oil and wastes your products.

Nice-to-Have Equipment

If you find you want to make fancier products with lots of ingredients, or if you want to package your products beautifully for gift-giving or sale, these tools are fantastic to add your supply stash.

Aromatherapy inhalers: These can be purchased in bulk, and many are reusable.

Aromatherapy jewelry: If you wear jewelry, you may enjoy adding an aromatherapy pendant or bracelet to your collection. These items are reusable and come in a variety of styles.

Double boiler: This is an excellent tool for melting waxes and crafting your own skin creams.

Essential oil dispensing syringes: Purpose-built for essential oils or medical use, these syringes are measured in milliliters (ml).

Essential oil key tool: Removing roller balls and orifice reducers from essential oil bottles can be a challenge; this tool makes an otherwise frustrating process fast and easy.

Glass eye droppers or pipettes: Perfect for pulling essential oils from larger wholesale-size bottles, pipettes and droppers help you measure drops precisely.

Glass roller bottles: These containers are wonderful for holding liquid lip balms, soothing temple rubs, perfumes, and much more.

Lip balm filling tray: If you want to make lots of lip balm and store it in handy tubes, you'll love how a filling tray makes the process quick, simple, and relatively mess-free.

Mixer: A handheld or stand mixer is good for whipping up rich body creams and blending big batches of product.

Specialty containers: Items such as tins, lip balm tubes, and cosmetics jars give your products a beautiful, finished look.

Storage bag or box: An insulated bag or box offers the ideal solution for protecting your essential oils from heat and light.

Carrier Oils

Carrier oils are used to dilute essential oils and prevent them from irritating your skin. There are many different types available; here are a few of the most popular. If you want to save money, use light olive oil or sunflower seed oil, which can be found at the supermarket.

Avocado oil: You can make your massage oils richer by adding a little avocado oil. This oil is very heavy and absorbs slowly; it has a strong fragrance, which you may or may not like.

Coconut oil: A unique oil that's solid above 76 degrees, coconut oil is ideal for making simple balms and lotions that melt when applied to skin. It is highly moisturizing and rich in vitamin E, plus it offers antibacterial and antifungal activity. Fractionated coconut oil has been processed to remain in a liquid state and is fantastic for making massage oils and more.

Fractionated coconut oil: Unlike virgin coconut oil, this product has no odor, and it remains in a liquid state. It penetrates very quickly and leaves just a trace of oil behind on the skin.

Jojoba oil: This oil is more expensive than many other carrier oils; but, its long shelf life and excellent absorption make it a favorite. If you suffer from acne or have very oily skin, you might consider replacing other carriers with this one, or blending it to give your carrier oil a lighter feel.

Rosehip oil: This is another expensive carrier oil, but it's one that's well worth adding to your apothecary. It is high in antioxidants, and it makes a fantastic addition to skin care products, especially for those hoping to age as gracefully as possible. A little goes a long way; you can blend it with other carriers and still reap the benefits.

Sweet almond oil: Sourced from almond kernels, this oil offers a very light, nutty fragrance. It absorbs quickly and leaves just a trace of oil behind.

Helpful Ingredients

Many recipes in this book require additional ingredients, such as witch hazel, unscented body wash, unscented lotion, Epsom salts, and more. Many of these ingredients can be purchased at the supermarket, while others are found online or at health food stores. This is not an exhaustive list, but it will help you stock up so you're ready to make a variety of recipes.

Aloe vera gel: Aloe gel is an excellent base for quick, natural moisturizers. It dilutes essential oils beautifully, and gives body care products a light, fresh feel. Use a clear, unscented type.

Baking soda: Some body care recipes and household cleaners call for this basic ingredient. Buy a big box and get ready to have fun with it.

Beeswax: Beeswax stiffens balms beautifully, while sealing in moisture. You can use a vegan alternative if you like; candelilla wax, carnauba wax, and organic soy wax are suitable stand-ins.

Butters: Shea, mango, and cocoa butters are essential for making thick, rich body butters that offer outstanding hydration. Each has a distinct texture and odor.

Castile soap: You can make a variety of household cleaners with castile soap, just use the unscented variety. You can save money by purchasing a bar, grating it, and then dissolving it in two quarts of boiling water before cooling it and pouring it into jars for storage. This is a little labor-intensive but it'll help you save money on a nice, natural base for your products.

Epsom salts: Many remedies call for a soothing aromatherapy bath. Epsom salts are the perfect medium for getting essential oils into your bath without leaving a messy ring behind.

Unscented body wash, shampoo, conditioner, and lotion: While you can make your own basic, unscented body care products, for simplicity this book makes extensive use of unscented bases. These are least expensive when purchased in bulk online.

Virgin coconut oil: Often subbing for shortening in your kitchen, this is fantastic for oil pulling and dental health recipes, and it makes its way into a variety of balms and moisturizers, too.

White vinegar: Don't let the sour smell prevent you from trying the many household recipes that call for white vinegar. Its odor evaporates quickly, leaving your home smelling of your favorite essential oils.

Witch hazel: This herbal tonic lets you make lovely skin toners, refreshing body sprays, and other products. It's inexpensive and very easy to find at drugstores and most supermarkets. Look for the alcohol-free variety, which won't make dry skin worse.

Blending, Dilution, and Substitution Guides

Because essential oils are so powerful, it's important to understand how they should be blended, diluted, and substituted for one another. Here are the basics.

Creating Aromatherapy Blends

There are two goals for creating your own aromatherapy blends. The first is to enjoy a pleasurable personalized scent, and the second is to obtain therapeutic benefits for your body, mind, and spirit. Scent preferences are highly personal; what smells fantastic to some people repels others.

Resting Time

Combining your essential oils for a recipe, and then letting them rest—for as little as 1 hour, or up to 2 or 3 days—lets them blend and mingle chemically. This creates synergy and allows the aroma to fully develop. A good source of bottles for this purpose is to recycle your empty essential oil ones (cleaned and dried)—and it's good for the earth, too!

In general, oils from the same category (i.e., citrus, floral, herbal, or spice) tend to blend well with one another. You can't go wrong with a blend of lemon and grapefruit, for example, or with a combination of peppermint and rosemary. Citrus and spice oils tend to complement one another beautifully, and so do herbs and citrus; for example, many people enjoy the classic combination of lemon and peppermint.

When blending, you'll want to add your essential oils to one another first, allow them to mingle, and then add the carrier oil. Be sure to keep notes about your blends, so you can recreate or modify them later. If scent is your first priority, let those essential oils combine with one another for up to three days before deciding whether you like the scent, and before adding your carrier oil. The aroma often changes as the constituents blend with one another.

Beginners should get a feel for blending by using recipes before creating their own blends; it's best to familiarize yourself with the oils going into your blends so you know how strong they are. As you might guess, strongly scented oils such as clove and clary sage have a tendency to overpower lighter ones like lemon and grapefruit.

Using Oils Neat and in Dilutions

There are different opinions for how best to dilute essential oils, and whether it is ever safe to apply essential oils neat—that is, without diluting them first. Just like the subject of taking oils internally, neat application is a controversial topic with opinions that vary from one practitioner to the next. It is up to you to determine how best to apply your essential oils safely. The neat peppermint oil that I use to stop my migraines isn't appropriate for everyone; in someone with highly sensitive skin, it would probably cause some irritation.

The best way to avoid skin irritation or sensitization is to dilute your oils before using them. There are a few exceptions: Certain acute conditions can respond best to undiluted essential oils. A drop of undiluted lavender essential oil, for example, is an excellent treatment for a minor cut or scrape, while a drop of undiluted tea tree essential oil makes an outstanding treatment for foot fungus. These are just two of many instances when neat application can be highly beneficial. Certain oils are often used neat on acupressure points, too. In almost all cases though, the total amount is just 1 or 2 drops.

If you have sensitive skin, or want to treat an elder or a child under 12 with essential oils, it's a good idea to dilute even the oils generally considered safe for neat use before applying them. The same logic applies to women who are pregnant, people with serious illnesses, and anyone with a compromised immune system. Don't worry—the essential oil will still do its job; the carrier "carries" the essential oil into the skin, while acting as a buffer.

Remember, even when heavily diluted, certain oils are not safe for everyone. Check for contraindications before using an essential oil on anyone—especially if that person falls into one of the categories mentioned previously, such as a young child or elderly person.

When you blend essential oils with anything—a carrier oil, aloe vera gel, your bath water, or an unscented soap or lotion base for example—you're diluting it. Most topical treatments in this book are heavily diluted, but there are exceptions for certain first-aid applications, as well as other remedies.

General Dilution Guide: Create New Recipes Safely

Essential oil dilution isn't an exact science: Drop sizes differ depending on the essential oil's viscosity and the type of dropper used. Additionally, some essential oils are far stronger or "hotter" than others, and can require higher dilution rates—the percentage of essential oil relative to the percentage of carrier—for safety reasons as well as to ensure the scents aren't overpowering. Recipes often fall into gray areas, too. For example, a blend might contain between 1.5 and 2 percent essential oil to provide a balanced, pleasing scent, while offering a high level of safety.

For beginners ready to create new blends for topical use, the following basic dilution guidelines represent a roadmap. You can follow them exactly, or you can calculate how many drops of essential oil to use with a simple equation. Imagine you'd like to make just 1 teaspoon of a remedy that calls for 3 percent dilution. The following chart shows that a 3 percent dilution with 2 tablespoons (1 fluid ounce) of carrier oil calls for 24 drops of essential oil. Basic measurement guidelines tell you that 1 teaspoon is one-sixth of a fluid ounce: So, 24 divided by 6 is 4, meaning that 1 teaspoon of your remedy should contain 4 drops of essential oil.

Whenever you use a new essential oil, you'll find it helpful to conduct some research on recommended dilution rates. Since opinions about dilution tend to vary widely, it's often best to check a few sources before deciding how to proceed.

Essential oils are never safe for premature infants.

0.1 TO 0.2 PERCENT DILUTIONS

Dilutions between 0.1 and 0.2 percent are considered safe for infants up to 3 months old, so long as the infant was carried to full term and the oils used are considered safe for infants.

0.25 TO 0.5 PERCENT DILUTIONS

Dilutions between 0.25 and 0.5 percent are generally considered safe for full-term infants between 3 months and 24 months, so long as the oils used are considered safe for infants.

The 0.5 percent dilution is often appropriate for "hot" oils such as clove and thyme. This dilution rate is also considered safe for most infants up to 24 months, so long as the oils used are safe for this age range.

1 PERCENT DILUTION

The 1 percent dilution is usually appropriate for daily skin care products, as well as for individuals with sensitive skin. It is considered standard for children between the ages of 2 and 6 years, immunocompromised individuals, those with long-term health conditions, and elders. This dilution rate is also recommended for pregnant women, as long as the essential oils used are considered safe for use during pregnancy.

1.5 PERCENT DILUTION

The 1.5 percent dilution rate is considered standard for children between the ages of 6 years and 12 years, so long as the oils used are safe for this age range.

2 TO 2.5 PERCENT DILUTIONS

The 2 percent dilution rate is considered the *maximum* recommended rate for children between the ages of 2 years and 6 years, so long as the oils used are safe for this age range.

Dilutions between 2 and 2.5 percent are considered to be the standard for adult application.

3 PERCENT DILUTIONS AND HIGHER

The 3 percent dilution rate is considered the *maximum* for children between the ages of 6 years and 12 years so long as the oils used are safe for this age range.

Higher percentage rates are usually indicated for treating acute conditions over a short period, on a relatively small part of the body. Insect repellents, hand sanitizers, perfumes, and household products tend to contain higher percentages as well. Feel free to dilute them further if you like; experimentation will help you determine whether lower dilutions meet your needs.

Neat application is not represented in this chart. In general, small, spot treatments with a few oils like peppermint, eucalyptus, frankincense, tea tree, and lavender are considered safe, as are neat treatments for poison ivy, shingles, eczema, and other conditions that might involve larger areas of the skin, and that tend to respond well to neat application in their earliest, most irritated phases.

Remember: *Always check safety considerations when considering an essential oil for neat application.* Although a conservative approach may not seem terribly exciting, it is the safest.

Dilution Guide

This chart shows the number of drops of essential oil required for different dilution rates in varying amounts of carrier oils. If you need the carrier oil amount specified in ounces, see the measurement conversions chart on page 229.

DILUTION RATE	1 TABLESPOON CARRIER	2 TABLESPOONS CARRIER	¼ CUP CARRIER
0.25%	1 drop	2 drops	4 drops
0.5%	2 drops	4 drops	8 drops
1%	4 drops	8 drops	16 drops
1.5%	6 drops	12 drops	24 drops
2%	8 drops	16 drops	32 drops
2.5%	10 drops	20 drops	40 drops
3%	12 drops	24 drops	48 drops
4%	16 drops	32 drops	64 drops
5%	18 drops	36 drops	72 drops
10%	36 drops	72 drops	144 drops

¹/₂ CUP CARRIER	³/₄ CUP CARRIER	1 CUP CARRIER
8 drops	12 drops	16 drops
16 drops	24 drops	32 drops
32 drops	48 drops	64 drops
48 drops	72 drops	96 drops
64 drops	96 drops	128 drops
80 drops	120 drops	160 drops
96 drops	144 drops	192 drops
128 drops	192 drops	256 drops
144 drops	216 drops	288 drops
288 drops	432 drops	576 drops

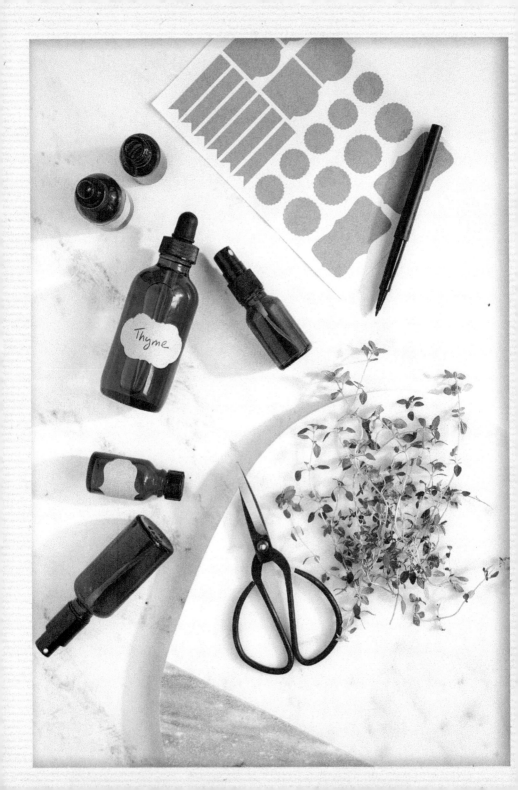

CHAPTER 3

Aromatherapy in Five Steps

While anyone can buy essential oils and start diffusing them immediately, learning in a systematic and methodical way can build a good foundation for those who want to dive deeper and explore aromatherapy safely. It doesn't take long to start integrating essential oils into your regular routine; all it requires is a bit of basic knowledge and a willingness to forgo the temporary pleasure of instant gratification.

Knowing what you want and need is step one. As in so many areas of life, you need a goal for your aromatherapy practice. Second, you want to avoid becoming overwhelmed when you shop for essential oils and start using them. Third, you want to avoid common pitfalls, as well as use your oils in the safest, most effective way possible. Simply put, you need to create a plan that works for you.

This simple five-step approach will help you do just that:

1. Determine your needs.
2. Go shopping.
3. Prepare your recipes.
4. Use your oils safely.
5. Store your oils well.

Let's look at each step in more detail.

Step 1: Determine Your Needs

What brings you to aromatherapy? What do you want to accomplish with your essential oils? These are two great questions to ask yourself to determine your needs, which will help you decide which essential oils to begin with. Some common reasons include:

- Treating common ailments naturally instead of with over-the-counter remedies

- Saving money on high-quality bath and body products

- Reducing household chemical use and saving money

- Interest in holistic health

If you're hoping to treat a specific ailment or two, you should research which essential oils are best for addressing your concerns. Whether you're looking for a way to increase energy naturally, enjoy better sleep, or get rid of tough headaches without reaching for pills, you'll find solutions in this book.

The same applies to other applications. Want a way to clean your home and do your laundry without worrying about potential problems listed on chemical warning labels? Look for essential oils that offer strong antibacterial properties and you'll be on your way to making effective, great-smelling household products.

For cosmetic concerns, research to see if an aromatherapy solution is available. The odds are high you'll find at least one that appeals to you—without the exorbitant price tags that typically accompany commercial preparations.

Once you've determined which issues you'd like to address, check the ingredients needed so you can buy your supplies before you get started. Whatever your goals, you'll soon discover that aromatherapy empowers you to improve your own health and handle some of life's little hiccups with ease. Once you know which oils you want to try first, and how little you actually need to get started, you're ready to take the next step.

Step 2: Go Shopping

You may feel tempted to buy all 15 oils in this book, and you might opt to do that if cost isn't a concern. However, if you're on a budget, use your goals to decide which ones are the highest priorities. You can simply make a list of oils from the list of "Must Haves" presented in chapter 1 (see page 15) to create a foundation for learning. If you aren't sure about your goals, or you just want to dip your toes in the water, I suggest you start with just one essential oil. Of all those available, lavender is the most versatile, with excellent benefits for your mind and body, such as the ability to help you get a naturally clean home, fresh-smelling laundry, and a good night's sleep.

Once you've started, and as finances allow, you can decide how you'd like to expand your collection. Maybe you've noticed a recipe that appeals to you and you're longing to try it. Perhaps you want to create some decadent bath salts or massage oil for yourself. Whatever the reason, use the following tips to select the best-quality essential oils at different price points.

- Decide if you want to shop locally or online

- Determine whether you want organic essential oils or conventional ones

- Consider how much money you need to get started (smaller bottles are less expensive and can make higher-quality oils more affordable)

- Check to be sure the essential oil is the only ingredient in the bottle, unless you are intentionally purchasing a prediluted product

- Read some reviews to see what others have to say

Step 3: Prepare Your Recipes

Read the recipe's ingredients and the instructions before you begin to be sure you have all the necessary tools, ingredients, and supplies. The recipes in this book are laid out in an easy-to-follow format, with practical tips for easy preparation.

If you're not sure you want to commit to creating the full quantity of a recipe because of the amount of essential oil it requires, prepare a smaller "test batch" by reducing the amount of each ingredient by half.

If you're new to aromatherapy, there are a few things to be aware of before you start formulating your first recipe. The following tips will ease your way and help you avoid some common pitfalls.

- Always conduct a patch test (see page 10) for each essential oil you plan to use before making a recipe. It is very disappointing to make a great-smelling massage oil and try it out, only to discover your skin is irritated by the blend you've created.

- Choose a clean, well-ventilated place to work. Your kitchen should do the trick.

- Make sure your tools are clean and dry before you start. Water can prevent your recipes from turning out the way you want them to.

- Sanitize and dry all containers before starting. Bacteria can spoil your remedies.

- Premeasure your ingredients so everything is ready to blend, especially if you're making a more complicated recipe, such as a body butter or lip balm.

- Be careful with your ingredients and cap your essential oils immediately after measuring your drops. This will prevent spills as well as keep your oils from evaporating.

- Keep little ones occupied, or make your recipes while they're napping.

- Slow-moving essential oil won't drip? Hold your bottle at an angle instead of straight up and down. It might take a few seconds, but the oil will flow with just a bit of patience.

- Have an empty essential oil bottle? You can make a nice linen mist or body spray by warming about 2 cups of water and letting your essential bottle soak in it for at least 10 minutes. Bottle the water and enjoy it. Be sure to save your bottles for refilling later.

Step 4: Use Your Oils Safely

Essential oils are natural, but they're also extremely powerful. It's important to approach working with them respectfully. If essential oil gets into your eyes, flush them continuously with a saline solution. If an oil gets onto mucus membranes, immediately flush the area with vegetable oil or cold milk (not water). Always seek medical attention if discomfort persists.

You learned some basic safety measures in chapter 2 (see page 31); answers to more in-depth safety questions are found here.

Q: HOW OFTEN CAN I DIFFUSE?

A: It's fine to diffuse essential oils daily, but it's a good idea to rotate oils throughout the week to avoid sensitization.

Q: CAN I USE DIFFERENT ESSENTIAL OILS FOR DIFFERENT NEEDS ALL AT THE SAME TIME?

A: You can use multiple essential oils throughout the day, but pace yourself. You should give each oil enough time to do its job. If you're using heavily diluted essential oils in bath and beauty products, it's fine to enjoy them one after another as you would normally do with other body products.

Q: IS IT POSSIBLE TO USE TOO MUCH ESSENTIAL OIL?

A: Yes: Unless you're treating an acute condition over a period of several days, you should use no more than 3 to 4 drops of each essential oil over the course of a given day, and you shouldn't use strong topical solutions unless necessary. Overuse can lead to allergies and hypersensitivity. If this happens, you'll get an unpleasant reaction each time you use the oil in the future.

Q: SHOULD I TAKE A BREAK FROM MY ESSENTIAL OILS?

A: It's fine to use highly diluted oils daily—for example, in soaps and shampoos. If you've been using stronger remedies, give your body a one-week break for every two weeks of topical essential oil use.

Q: SHOULD I SWITCH APPLICATION SITES TO AVOID SENSITIZATION?

A: Yes, if you tend to use the same oil over and over again, and particularly if you use oils neat. Overuse can cause rashes, and in some cases serious skin irritation can develop.

Step 5: Store Your Oils Well

Storing essential oils properly preserves their therapeutic properties. While essential oils don't go rancid the same way carriers can, they are subject to oxidization when exposed to heat and light. Citrus oils start to lose their potency about six months after opening, so make use of them when they're at their freshest. The good news is, when properly stored, most essential oils have a shelf life of at least one year, and many will stay fresh for two years or longer. Some, such as patchouli, actually improve with age.

Safety Tips for the Entire Household

- Keep essential oils and remedies out of reach of children and pets.
- Read all warning labels.
- Learn about each new essential oil before using it.
- If you take prescription medications, have a chronic illness, or have a compromised immune system, check with a knowledgeable practitioner before using essential oils. Certain oils may be contraindicated.
- Contact poison control and seek immediate medical treatment for a child who has consumed essential oil. Take the bottle when you go to the emergency department.
- Always conduct patch tests before using new essential oils.
- Keep essential oils away from flames and heat sources.
- Avoid getting essential oils in your eyes and mucus membranes.
- Do not put essential oil in your ears.
- Always wash your hands after using essential oils.
- Wear gloves when using household cleaners for an extended length of time.

The best way to store your essential oils is to keep them in a cool, dark area with a stable temperature. An insulated case is ideal, and a padded cooler can do the trick. Never store your essential oils in direct sunlight, as this causes rapid deterioration.

Once blended, most remedies keep for about six months, depending on the ingredients and the storage conditions. Make small batches if to avoid waste, or share your products with others. Refrigeration can greatly extend shelf life, too.

It's time to replace your oils and blends when their scents weaken or start to smell a bit off. Your nose is an excellent tool for detecting oils that are no longer suitable for aromatherapy.

Troubleshooting Questions

Q: MY DIFFUSER ISN'T WORKING PROPERLY. IS THERE A SOLUTION?

A: Check the manufacturer's guidelines for cleaning. Be sure to unplug your diffuser before servicing it.

Q: I'M TILTING MY ESSENTIAL OIL BUT IT STILL REFUSES TO DRIP.

A: Try warming the essential oil bottle in your hands for 30 to 60 seconds. If stubbornness persists, remove the orifice reducer and carefully measure the oil for your recipe.

Q: I HAVE VERY SENSITIVE SKIN AND I CAN'T USE TOPICAL REMEDIES. CAN I STILL USE ESSENTIAL OILS?

A: You can try inhalation methods that don't put your skin in direct contact with essential oil vapors; diffusion may be suitable. Start with just 1 drop of essential oil at a time to see how you respond. Be sure to wear gloves when dispensing your essential oil. Stop use immediately if you feel uncomfortable, and seek medical attention if discomfort persists.

Q: I DON'T HAVE THE EXACT CARRIER RECOMMENDED IN A RECIPE. CAN I TRY A DIFFERENT ONE?

A: Yes, carriers are interchangeable. Some, such as rosehip and calendula oils, have beneficial properties that improve the recipes they're used in. Feel free to substitute, but your results might be different than those made with the original recipe.

Q: I BOUGHT ESSENTIAL OIL BUT IT DOESN'T HAVE AN ORIFICE REDUCER FOR "DROPPING" THE OIL FROM THE BOTTLE. WHAT CAN I DO?

A: You can purchase a package of orifice reducers from a store that carries essential oil supplies. Several options are available online.

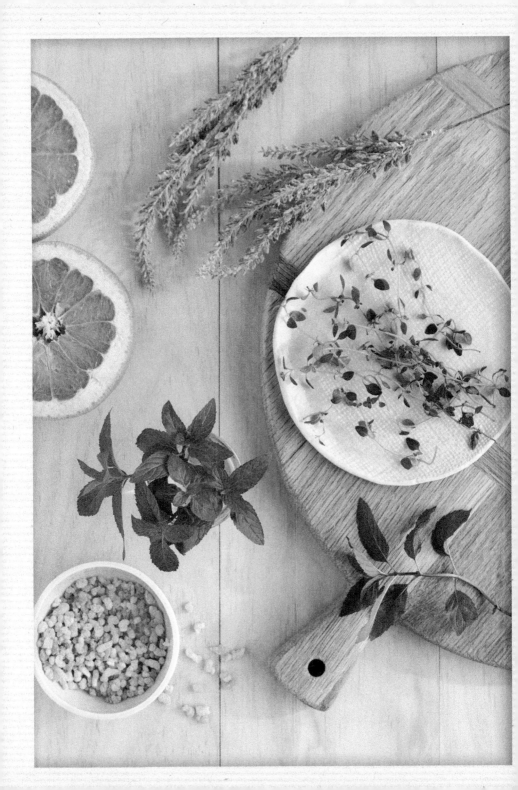

Profiles of Essential Oil All-Stars

I t's so easy to find aromatherapy products these days! While accessibility is high on my list of positives, this means that some curious consumers end up using essential oils without knowing what they're doing—which can open them, and their loved ones up to the potential for skin irritation and allergic responses. Although these problems can be minor, it's best to protect yourself by exploring aromatherapy safely.

Fifteen Essential Oil Profiles

Knowledge is key to safe essential oil use. The following profiles offer a well-rounded look at the 15 essential oils showcased in this book, providing you with each oil's Latin name, its description, and important safety information. You'll also learn about opportunities for blending each essential oil with others, and you'll discover which healing properties it possesses. Finally, you will discover some of the most common ways to enjoy and use each of these essential oils.

Each description also includes notes on substituting essential oils. Before substituting, ask yourself why you want to use the oil in question, and check substitutes for similar properties.

Clary Sage

SALVIA SCLAREA

BLENDS WELL WITH

Bergamot
Cedarwood
Clove
Lemon
Geranium
German chamomile
Juniper berry
Frankincense
Ginger
Grapefruit
Lavender
Patchouli
Peppermint
Roman chamomile
Sandalwood
Sweet orange
Tea tree
Vitex berry

SUBSTITUTE WITH

Anise seed
Bergamot
Fennel
Frankincense
Lavender
Red mandarin
Rosemary
Sandalwood
Tarragon

If you want an essential oil to ease PMS or menopause symptoms, you'll appreciate what clary sage can do for you. This versatile oil makes short work of common complaints ranging from hormone-induced mood swings to painful, period-related cramping, thanks to a constituent called *sclareol*; it offers a structure similar to that of estrogen, and, for many women, it helps promote a sense of balanced calm. Clary sage shines in soothing bedtime formulas, too, and makes an uplifting addition to any mood-boosting regimen. Most people like the scent of clary sage; it is comforting, herbaceous, and promotes a relaxed atmosphere.

Precautions

- **Avoid clary sage essential oil during pregnancy.** It is a strong emmenagogue that can promote uterine contractions.

- Do not use topically on children under age 6 years.

- Clary sage essential oil can promote drowsiness. Do not use it before driving, or while operating machinery.

- Do not use clary sage essential oil in combination with alcohol.

- If taking prescription drugs, check with your doctor before adding clary sage to your regimen.

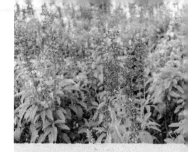

Application Methods

INHALATION: Try adding 3 drops of clary sage to an essential oil inhaler or placing 1 or 2 drops on your pillowcase just before lying down. If adding it to a diffuser, use the number of drops recommended by the diffuser's manufacturer.

TOPICAL: Use blends containing clary sage as a soothing temple rub or massage oil. This method is ideal for relaxation and meditation.

BATH: Bath salts, body washes, hair products, and bath oils let you enjoy clary sage for its emotionally grounding effects as well as its ability to nourish and balance skin and hair.

Popular Uses

- Clary sage promotes an almost instant sense of calm, so it's ideal to use in relaxing blends for dealing with stress or anxiety, or try using it on its own.

- Since clary sage can help bring troubled hormones back into balance, it makes an excellent treatment for PMS and menopause symptoms, such as mood swings and hot flashes. Used in a massage blend, it eases period pain.

HEALING PROPERTIES

Antidepressant
Antiseptic
Antispasmodic
Aphrodisiac
Astringent
Bactericidal
Carminative
Deodorant
Digestive
Emmenagogue
Euphoric
Hypotensive
Nervine
Sedative
Stomachic

IDEAL FOR TREATING

Anxiety
Body odor
Depression
Emotional upset
Exhaustion
Insomnia
Menopause symptoms
Painful periods
PMS
Stress

Clove

SYZYGIUM AROMATICUM

Like the popular spice from which it is derived, clove essential oil has a sweet, spicy scent that can boost your mood in seconds. Its warm, welcoming fragrance makes it ideal for creating natural air-freshening blends to scent your home. Clove is also outstanding as a pain reliever, so much so that dentists used it on their patients before contemporary numbing agents became available. It is still found in some toothpastes and over-the-counter toothache remedies. Clove is an outstanding addition to blends for easing muscle and joint pain, and it can help with indigestion.

BLENDS WELL WITH

Allspice
Basil
Benzoin
Bergamot
Cinnamon
Clary sage
Ginger
Grapefruit
Helichrysum
Hops
Lavender
Lemon
Lime
Orange
Peppermint
Rosemary
Sandalwood
Sweet orange
Ylang-ylang
Yuzu

SUBSTITUTE WITH

Cinnamon
German chamomile
Ginger
Nutmeg
Oregano
Patchouli
Roman chamomile
Tea tree
Thyme

Precautions

- Clove is a "hot" essential oil and it *must be diluted* for all applications except toothaches.
- **Avoid clove essential oil during pregnancy.**
- Do not use clove essential oil if you suffer from liver or kidney disease.

Application Methods

INHALATION: Mixed into 1 cup of water, a few drops of clove essential oil make a quick, uplifting room spray. If adding it to a diffuser,

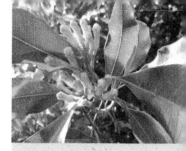

use the number of drops recommended by the diffuser's manufacturer.

TOPICAL: Try adding 1 or 2 drops of clove essential oil to 1 teaspoon of your favorite carrier oil for an instant, warming massage. It's ideal for post-workout blends and comforting rubs to ease coughs and congestion during cold and flu season.

BATH: Bath salts, body washes, hair products, and bath oils let you take advantage of clove's enticing, mood-boosting fragrance, either on its own or with other essential oils.

Popular Uses

- Bugs hate clove, so it's excellent as a natural insect repellent. Mix it with borax or diatomaceous earth to create an insect barrier around your home's foundation, and try it in a personal insect-repellent blend next time you want mosquitoes to leave you alone.

- Replace expensive over-the-counter dental products with clove essential oil. If you have a toothache and the dentist can't see you right away, add 1 drop of clove essential oil to a cotton ball and press it to the sore tooth.

- Clove has antifungal, antiviral, and antiseptic properties, making it an excellent addition to purifying blends for keeping your home clean naturally. It's even listed in many of the most popular recipes for traditional Thieves disinfecting blends.

HEALING PROPERTIES

Analgesic
Antifungal
Antiseptic
Antispasmodic
Antiviral
Aphrodisiac
Carminative
Disinfectant
Insecticide
Insect repellent
Stimulant
Stomachic

IDEAL FOR TREATING

Acne
Athlete's foot
Bad breath
Body odor
Bruises
Cold and flu care
Cramping
Headache
Indigestion
Insect bites and bee stings
Jock itch
Muscle pain
Nail fungus
Ringworm
Sinusitis
Toothache

Eucalyptus

EUCALYPTUS GLOBULUS

BLENDS WELL WITH

Benzoin

Cajuput

Lavender

Lemon

Lemongrass

Pine

Rosemary

Tea Tree

Thyme

SUBSTITUTE WITH

Eucalyptus radiata

Lavender

Peppermint

Tea Tree

Known for its fresh, invigorating fragrance, eucalyptus essential oil is a fantastic addition to household cleaners and natural air fresheners. Its pain-relieving and antiseptic qualities make it an important ingredient in many natural first-aid remedies. Additionally, eucalyptus has the ability to reduce mucus membrane swelling and is among the best essential oils for treating cold and flu symptoms. Most insects dislike eucalyptus, so it is also an effective addition to natural insect repellents.

Precautions

- Do not use topically on children under age 6 years.
- Do not use eucalyptus essential oil if you have epilepsy.
- Do not use eucalyptus essential oil if you have high blood pressure.
- Use eucalyptus in moderation; excessive use can contribute to headaches.

Application Methods

INHALATION: Mixed with water, eucalyptus essential oil makes a quick, uplifting room spray or shower cleaner. Place 3 drops in an essential oil inhaler to assist with cold and flu symptoms. If adding it to a diffuser, use the number of drops recommended by the diffuser's manufacturer.

TOPICAL: Try adding 4 to 6 drops of eucalyptus essential oil to 1 tablespoon of your favorite carrier oil for soothing relief from insect bites and other minor wounds.

BATH: Bath salts, body washes, hair products, and bath oils let you take advantage of eucalyptus's refreshing fragrance, either on its own or with other essential oils. A warm bath scented with eucalyptus can provide relief from cold and flu symptoms.

Popular Uses

- Eucalyptus helps compromised skin heal faster, so it's useful for treating rashes, sunburns, and more. If you've spent too long in the sun, try blending 30 drops of eucalyptus with ½ cup of aloe gel. Use just enough to lightly coat the burned areas.

- As eucalyptus is a febrifuge, you can use it in remedies to help control fevers. Try mixing 15 drops of eucalyptus essential oil with 5 drops of peppermint essential oil, and add ½ cup of water. Lightly mist your body every 1 to 2 hours until your temperature returns to normal. This mixture also offers some cool relief from hot weather.

- Thanks to its antibacterial, antimicrobial, and antiseptic properties, eucalyptus makes an effective addition to household cleaners.

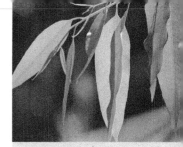

HEALING PROPERTIES

Analgesic
Antibacterial
Anti-inflammatory
Antiseptic
Antispasmodic
Antiviral
Astringent
Cicatrizant
Decongestant
Deodorant
Depurative
Diuretic
Expectorant
Febrifuge
Rubefacient
Stimulant
Vermifuge
Vulnerary

IDEAL FOR TREATING

Asthma
Blisters
Burns
Cold and flu care
Congestion
Cuts and scrapes
Headaches
Insect bites and
   bee stings
Sinusitis
Sunburn

Frankincense

BOSWELLIA CARTERII, B. SERRATA, B. SACRA

BLENDS WELL WITH

Bergamot
Black pepper
Cinnamon
Clove
Cypress
Geranium
Grapefruit
Helichrysum
Lavender
Lemon
Mandarin
Neroli
Orange
Palmarosa
Patchouli
Pine
Rose
Rose geranium
Vetiver
Ylang-ylang

SUBSTITUTE WITH

Galbanum
Helichrysum
Myrrh
Palo santo
Patchouli
Sandalwood

Many are familiar with frankincense—it's one of the three gifts the Magi brought to the infant Jesus in the nativity story. It's warm, woody scent with a touch of spice makes it a classic incense ingredient. Besides offering a deep, calming influence, frankincense is a versatile essential oil with benefits for the skin, respiratory tract, and more.

Precautions

○ **Do not use during pregnancy, or while breastfeeding.**

Application Methods

INHALATION: Mixed into 1 cup of water and misted into the air, a few drops of frankincense essential oil create a peaceful, meditative feeling. If adding it to a diffuser, use the number of drops recommended by the diffuser's manufacturer.

TOPICAL: Add 9 drops of frankincense essential oil to 1 tablespoon of your favorite carrier oil for a relaxing moisturizer you can use all over.

BATH: Use frankincense with clary sage and lavender for a calming bedtime treat. You can add a few drops of each essential oil to your bathwater, or create a special blend to scent lotion or body oil.

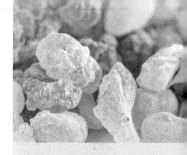

Popular Uses

◦ Frankincense is safe for babies, and it's well-known for its ability to heal rashes. Try blending 6 drops of frankincense essential oil with 2 tablespoons (1 ounce) of melted lanolin for a protective, all-natural diaper balm. A little dab—about ½ teaspoon—provides a soothing moisture barrier.

◦ Enhance your meditation practice by diffusing frankincense. Its relaxing fragrance and mild sedative quality combine to enhance your ability to breathe deeply and let go of stress.

◦ If you're coming down with a cold, add 3 drops of frankincense essential oil to an aromatherapy inhaler and use it to ease congestion. As a natural expectorant, it can help keep your airways clear.

HEALING PROPERTIES

Antiseptic
Astringent
Carminative
Cicatrizant
Cytophylactic
Digestive
Diuretic
Emmenagogue
Expectorant
Sedative
Vulnerary

IDEAL FOR TREATING

Asthma
Bronchitis
Cold and flu symptoms
Colic
Gas
Inflammation
Laryngitis
Minor cuts and scrapes
Rashes
Scars

Geranium

PELARGONIUM ODORATISSIMUM

BLENDS WELL WITH

Atlas cedar
Bergamot
Carrot seed
Cedarwood
Clary sage
Cucumber seed
German chamomile
Grapefruit
Helichrysum
Jasmine
Juniper berry
Lavender
Lemon
Lemongrass
Lime
Melissa
Roman chamomile
Rosemary

SUBSTITUTE WITH

Rose geranium

If you enjoy natural skin care products, you may have seen geranium listed on some you've tried. This is because it has several properties that benefit dry, itchy, aging skin. And geranium essential oil offers gentle, hormone-balancing benefits for women who want relief from PMS and menopause symptoms. One of geranium's constituents, *geraniol,* is a top ingredient in many natural insect repellents; if you'd like to make your own bug spray, geranium is an excellent addition.

Precautions

- Geranium can reduce blood sugar; it is not recommended for diabetics.
- **Do not use during pregnancy.**

Application Methods

INHALATION: Mixed into 1 cup of rosewater, a few drops of geranium essential oil can create a romantic atmosphere. In an essential oil inhaler or aromatherapy jewelry, its scent is both uplifting and refreshing. If adding geranium to a diffuser, use the number of drops recommended by the diffuser's manufacturer.

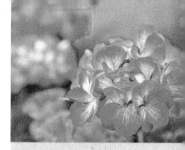

TOPICAL: Try adding 6 to 8 drops of geranium essential oil to 1 teaspoon of your favorite carrier oil for a quick, nourishing massage oil that works wonders for dry skin.

BATH: Feeling stressed? Try creating a blend with geranium, Roman chamomile, and lavender to add to your bath and body products. These oils go very well together; try different proportions of each to find a scent that appeals to you.

Popular Uses

- Because geranium essential oil nourishes and heals skin, it's found in a variety of facial, bath, and body products. Classic recipes call for the addition of rose essential oil, too. If you'd like to experiment with this combination and maintain your budget, look for prediluted rose essential oil, which is available at different concentrations. Some companies offer pure rose essential oil in sample sizes, too.

- All hair types benefit from geranium essential oil. You can make your own shampoo and conditioner with unscented bases, or you can mix 15 drops of geranium essential oil with ½ cup of water for a quick leave-in spray.

- While geranium is classified as a floral essential oil, its aroma has a crisp, green edge that makes it fantastic for freshening air. Alone or blended with a citrus oil such as lemon or grapefruit, geranium helps your home smell fantastic, while providing some stress-relieving aromatherapy benefits.

HEALING PROPERTIES

Antiseptic
Astringent
Cicatrizant
Cytophylactic
Diuretic
Deodorant
Hemostatic
Styptic
Tonic
Vermifuge
Vulnerary

IDEAL FOR TREATING

Aging skin
Anxiety
Combination skin
Dry skin
Eczema
Menopause symptoms
Mild postnatal depression
Mood swings
PMS symptoms
Shingles
Stress

Grapefruit

CITRUS PARADISI, C. RACEMOSE,
C. MAXIMA VAR. RACEMOSA

BLENDS WELL WITH

Bergamot
Cardamom
Cedarwood
Cinnamon
Clove
Coriander
Cypress
Geranium
German Chamomile
Ginger
Juniper berry
Lavender
Lemon
Lime
Mandarin
Patchouli
Peppermint
Red mandarin
Roman chamomile
Yuzu

SUBSTITUTE WITH

Bergamot
Lemon
Lime
Orange
Red mandarin
Tangerine
Yuzu

Whenever I'm tired or in a funk, I reach for citrus; grapefruit happens to be one of the best mood-boosting oils there is. Its sweet, refreshing scent has a pleasant tangy note, perfect for creating a cheerful atmosphere in your home or office while helping to purify the air, as well as to contribute antibacterial action to cleaning solutions. Besides its marvelous psychological bene-fits, grapefruit is an excellent remedy for water retention. And those watching their waistlines enjoy its ability to take the mind off bothersome food cravings.

Precautions

- Do not use if you take statins or other medications that interact with grapefruit.

- Grapefruit is phototoxic and can increase the likelihood of sunburn. Do not expose treated areas to direct sunlight for 12 hours after use.

Application Methods

INHALATION: Added to an essential oil inhaler or aromatherapy pendant, 3 or 4 drops of grapefruit essential oil can help you stay focused when working or studying. If adding it to a diffuser, use the number of drops recom-mended by the diffuser's manufacturer.

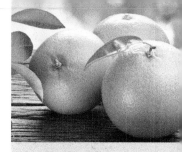

TOPICAL: Combine 4 drops of grapefruit essential oil with 1 teaspoon of your favorite carrier oil for a quick, detoxifying massage.

BATH: If you're looking for an uplifting, energizing addition to your bath and body care lineup, create blends that include grapefruit. It's fantastic in everything from basic bath salts to invigorating sugar scrubs.

Popular Uses

○ Like other citrus oils, grapefruit is good for eliminating odors and sanitizing surfaces. Mix it into household cleansers with complementary essential oils for fresher bathrooms, kitchens, and more.

○ For swollen feet and legs, create a massage blend with 6 drops of grapefruit essential oil per teaspoon of carrier oil. Use it as often as you'd like to support circulation and help reduce water retention.

○ Grapefruit offers good antimicrobial properties, and is an effective addition to first-aid remedies for minor wounds.

HEALING PROPERTIES

Antibacterial
Antidepressant
Antiseptic
Aperitif
Astringent
Digestive
Disinfectant
Diuretic
Lymphatic stimulant
Tonic

IDEAL FOR TREATING

Acne
Anxiety
Cellulite
Depression
Hangover
Headache
Fatigue
Food cravings
Menstrual cramps
Mood swings
Muscle cramps
Muscle pain
Oily skin
Stress
Water retention

Lavender

LAVANDULA ANGUSTIFOLIA

BLENDS WELL WITH

Bergamot
Black pepper
Cedarwood
Clary sage
Clove
Cypress
Eucalyptus
Frankincense
Geranium
German chamomile
Grapefruit
Lemon
Lemongrass
Patchouli
Peppermint
Roman chamomile
Rosemary
Tea Tree
Thyme
Vetiver

SUBSTITUTE WITH

Eucalyptus
Frankincense
German chamomile
Helichrysum
Hyssop
Lavandin
Patchouli
Roman chamomile
Tea tree

Lavender is renowned for its ability to calm and quiet the mind, while promoting a sense of deep relaxation. Its usefulness in first-aid treatments is near-legendary thanks to its healing and regenerative properties, and it's a valuable addition to bath and body products and household cleaners. It is an enormously versatile essential oil, so if you're looking for a single oil to start with, lavender provides an outstanding introduction to aromatherapy.

Precautions

○ Overuse can cause allergic reactions, especially with neat application. Use lavender judiciously, even though it is generally regarded as safe.

Application Methods

INHALATION: Lavender is a gentle, but effective remedy for stuffy sinuses; inhaling it provides relief while soothing inflamed nasal linings. If adding it to a diffuser, use the number of drops recommended by the diffuser's manufacturer.

TOPICAL: One of a few essential oils safe for undiluted use, lavender quickly takes the sting out of a minor burn, cut, or scrape. Drip a single drop onto the affected area after cleansing and allow it to air-dry.

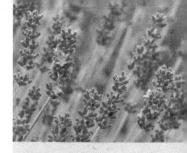

BATH: Try making your own bath and beauty products that take advantage of lavender's comforting fragrance. It's ideal for using on its own and, because it blends beautifully with many other essential oils, the sky really is the limit!

Popular Uses

- Whip up a quick linen spray by adding 10 drops of lavender essential oil to 1 cup of water. Lightly spritz your sheets, comforter, and pillows at bedtime. This spray doubles as an all-natural air freshener.

- Lavender is both an antibacterial and antiviral agent, so it's ideal for adding to household cleaners. One versatile spray can help you keep a variety of surfaces clean.

- Because most people like its fragrance, it makes a wonderful addition to homemade gifts; scented sachets, potpourri, and bath salts are just a few favorites.

HEALING PROPERTIES

Analgesic
Antidepressant
Anti-inflammatory
Antiseptic
Antispasmodic
Antiviral
Bactericide
Carminative
Cholagogue
Cicatrizant
Cordial
Cytophylactic
Decongestant
Deodorant
Diuretic
Hypotensive
Nervine
Rubefacient
Sedative
Sudorific
Vulnerary

IDEAL FOR TREATING

Anxiety
Depression
Insect bites
Insomnia
Minor burns
Minor cuts
 and scrapes
Sunburns

Lemon

CITRUS LIMONUM

BLENDS WELL WITH

Allspice
Benzoin
Caraway seed
Cardamom
Clove
Eucalyptus
Fennel seed
Frankincense
Geranium
Ginger
Grapefruit
Lavender
Lemongrass
Orange
Patchouli
Peppermint
Rosemary
Tangerine
Tea tree
Thyme

SUBSTITUTE WITH

Grapefruit
Mandarin
Orange
Red mandarin
Yuzu

Crisp, refreshing, and delightfully tangy, lemon essential oil is like sunshine in a bottle. As with other citrus oils, it can give your mood a much-needed boost when you're feeling dreary, and if your energy level is lagging, a whiff of lemon can help you feel more alert. This versatile oil really shines in household cleaners; so much so that many commercial products contain it.

Precautions

- Lemon essential oil is phototoxic and can increase the likelihood of sunburn. Do not expose treated areas to direct sunlight for 12 hours after use.

Application Methods

INHALATION: Blend 15 to 20 drops of lemon essential oil with 1 cup of water for a quick room spray that eliminates stale odors and creates a cheerful atmosphere. If adding it to a diffuser, use the number of drops recommended by the diffuser's manufacturer.

TOPICAL: Try adding 1 or 2 drops of lemon essential oil to a eucalyptus, tea tree, or rosemary blend and dilute with your favorite carrier oil for a comforting anticongestion blend to use during cold or allergy season. Remember to keep treated areas out of direct sunlight.

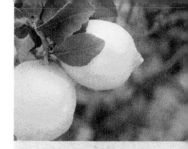

BATH: Bath and body products treat you to lemon's luscious fragrance, while treating your mood to an instant boost. Lemon is nice on its own, with other citrus oils, and with a wide variety of other spicy- or herbal-scented oils.

Popular Uses

- Lemon is a top ingredient in DIY cleaning solutions for everything from the kitchen to the bathroom. It's an excellent anti-bacterial and antiseptic agent, plus its fragrance is versatile enough to blend with a wide variety of other essential oils. If you're ready to experiment with your own household cleaning blends, you'll probably enjoy adding lemon.

- Lemon is a scent that just about everyone likes, and its ability to create a cheerful atmosphere is well known. Diffusing lemon alone or with other citrus essential oils is a great way to make your entire house smell clean, while treating yourself to some wonderful psychological benefits.

- Lemon's antiseptic and bactericidal actions make it an ally during cold and flu season. Try adding 3 drops to an essential oil inhaler next time you have a cough or cold symptoms. If your doctor approves, use it to soothe your symptoms while prescription antibiotics work behind the scenes.

HEALING PROPERTIES

Antifungal
Antiseptic
Bactericidal
Carminative
Cicatrizant
Depurative
Diaphoretic
Diuretic
Febrifuge
Hemostatic
Hypotensive
Insecticidal
Rubefacient
Tonic
Vermifuge

IDEAL FOR TREATING

Allergies
Asthma
Athlete's foot
Bronchitis
Congestion
Emotional upset
Jock itch
Nail fungus
Respiratory infections
Ringworm
Stress

Lemongrass

CYMBOPOGON CITRATUS, C. FLEXUOSUS

BLENDS WELL WITH

Basil
Cajuput
Cedarwood
Clary sage
Clove
Coriander
Cypress
Eucalyptus
Geranium
Ginger
Grapefruit
Lavender
Lemon
Patchouli
Peppermint
Rosemary
Tea Tree
Thyme

SUBSTITUTE WITH

Eucalyptus
Geranium
Lavender
Lemon
Tea tree

Lemongrass isn't just a popular kitchen herb; it's also the source of a versatile essential oil you can use for everything from soothing sore muscles, to keeping bugs from ruining outdoor fun. According to a study published in the *Libyan Journal of Medicine*, lemongrass exhibits strong antifungal action, even when confronted with a potent strain of yeast (*Candida albicans*). It also demonstrated strong anti-inflammatory action on irritated skin. The study's findings concluded that there is significant potential for the use of lemongrass in antifungal and anti-inflammatory drugs.

Precautions

- Do not use topically on children under age 2 years.
- Do not use on broken, irritated, or sensitive skin.

Application Methods

INHALATION: Mixed into 1 cup of water, 10 to 12 drops of lemongrass essential oil make a refreshing room spray that can help you focus. If adding lemongrass to a diffuser, use the number of drops recommended by the diffuser's manufacturer.

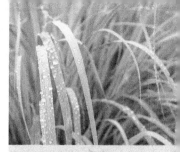

TOPICAL: Relieve joint pain by blending 5 drops of lemongrass essential oil with an equal amount of carrier oil.

BATH: Make a soak for sore muscles by blending 20 drops of lemongrass with 2 cups of Epsom salt. Spend 15 to 30 minutes relaxing and you'll emerge feeling light and refreshed.

Popular Uses

- A popular ingredient in insect repellents, lemongrass is even used in some commercial brands. Try it for yourself, either using lemongrass on its own or with other insect-repelling essential oils.

- Lemongrass is a traditional toothache remedy. Try it in mouthwash: Blend 6 drops lemongrass essential oil with 1 cup of water or vodka, and swish with about 2 teaspoons of the solution. Don't swallow this remedy; spit it out as you would a commercial mouth rinse.

- Many natural deodorant recipes call for lemongrass. Try it on its own or with other deodorizing essential oils.

HEALING PROPERTIES

Analgesic
Antidepressant
Antimicrobial
Antiseptic
Astringent
Bactericidal
Carminative
Deodorant
Diuretic
Febrifuge
Fungicidal
Insecticidal
Insect repellent
Nervine

IDEAL FOR TREATING

Athlete's foot
Headache
Jet lag
Jock itch
Nail fungus
Ringworm
Stress
Yeast infection

Patchouli

POGOSTEMON CABLIN

BLENDS WELL WITH

Bergamot
Cinnamon
Clary sage
Clove
Frankincense
Geranium
German chamomile
Ginger
Grapefruit
Lavender
Lemon
Lemongrass
Lime
Mandarin
Myrrh
Orange
Roman chamomile
Rosemary
Ylang-ylang
Yuzu

SUBSTITUTE WITH

Frankincense
Galbanum
Helichrysum
Hyssop
Lavender
Myrrh

Among the world's most popular perfume ingredients, patchouli has an intriguingly sweet scent with strong notes of wood and spice. Behind its remarkable fragrance lies a wide range of uses, beginning with its ability to repel insects. If you like spending time outdoors and want an alternative to commercial bug spray, create a blend with patchouli. The mosquitoes will leave you alone, even though you smell delightful. A little patchouli goes a long way, but don't worry about your bottle going bad—this is one essential oil that usually improves as it ages.

Precautions

- Generally regarded as safe

Application Methods

INHALATION: Mixed into 1 cup of water on its own or with a complementary essential oil, a few drops of patchouli make a delightful linen spray or natural perfume. If adding it to a diffuser, use the number of drops recommended by the diffuser's manufacturer.

TOPICAL: Try adding 3 or 4 drops of patchouli essential oil to 1 teaspoon of your favorite carrier oil for a relaxing massage blend.

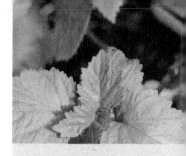

BATH: Patchouli essential oil can take basic blends such as lavender and rosemary to the next level. If you're feeling creative, make tiny batches of bath and body products to see what appeals to you.

Popular Uses

○ Patchouli is good for relieving stress, either on its own or with complementary essential oils such as peppermint. Some recipes call for using the oils undiluted; but if you have sensitive skin, use a carrier oil to prevent irritation.

○ For acne-prone and combination skin, patchouli offers soothing relief. Try blending 6 to 7 drops with ½ cup of witch hazel or micellar water and apply it liberally once or twice daily.

○ Dry and wrinkled skin benefit from patchouli, too; add 1 drop to your daily dose of facial moisturizer, blend it in with your finger, and apply as usual.

HEALING PROPERTIES

Antidepressant
Antiemetic
Antifungal
Anti-inflammatory
Antimicrobial
Antiseptic
Antiviral
Aphrodisiac
Astringent
Calmative
Carminative
Cicatrizant
Deodorant
Digestive
Diuretic
Febrifuge
Fungicidal
Insect repellent
Insecticide
Sedative

IDEAL FOR TREATING

Athlete's foot
Dandruff
Depression
Eczema
Hemorrhoids
Jock itch
Nail fungus
Ringworm
Yeast infection

Peppermint

MENTHA PIPERITA

BLENDS WELL
WITH

Basil
Benzoin
Black pepper
Catnip
Cypress
Eucalyptus
Geranium
German chamomile
Grapefruit
Juniper
Lavender
Lemon
Lemongrass
Niaouli
Orange
Pine
Rosemary
Spearmint
Tea Tree
Thyme

**SUBSTITUTE
WITH**

Catnip
Hyssop
Spearmint

If you suffer from tension headaches or migraines, you're likely to enjoy quick relief with just a few drops of peppermint essential oil. This refreshing essential oil offers a sweet, familiar fragrance once it is diffused, evaporated, or blended with a carrier oil. Some people can tolerate, or even enjoy, peppermint essential oil applied neat; others find the crisp, cold sensation uncomfortable, and very sensitive individuals suffer from severe irritation without dilution. It's very important to determine your tolerance level by testing it before use.

Precautions

- Can cause skin irritation, particularly in sensitive individuals.

- Overuse can lead to sensitization.

- Do not apply to mucus membranes; severe irritation can occur.

- **Do not use during pregnancy.**

- **Avoid if breastfeeding;** peppermint can decrease lactation. Note: If you are working to stop lactation after pregnancy or when weaning your baby, blend 15 to 20 drops of peppermint essential oil in 1 tablespoon of carrier oil and use a small amount to massage your breasts a few times per day. If you use this method, *do not* feed your breast milk to your infant.

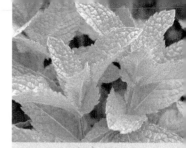

- Dilute heavily for use on infants and children under age 6 years. When using on young children and infants, do not apply peppermint to the face or chest area due to the risk of side effects when inhaling concentrated menthol present in the oil.

- Peppermint is an outstanding remedy for a variety of digestive complaints, but it can make heartburn worse.

Application Methods

INHALATION: Add 1 or 2 drops of peppermint essential oil to an aromatherapy inhaler or jewelry and take a few deep breaths to rid yourself of unwanted food cravings. If adding peppermint to a diffuser, use the number of drops recommended by the diffuser's manufacturer.

TOPICAL: Beat summer heat by blending 10 drops of peppermint with 1 cup of water in a misting bottle. Treat yourself to a light spritz for an instant cooling sensation.

BATH: Enjoy peppermint's invigorating scent in the shower. Simply apply a few drops of essential oil to a washcloth and place it on the shower floor. The vapors will rise up to greet your nose, and you'll emerge feeling refreshed.

Popular Uses

- Peppermint is such an effective breath freshener that it makes its way into a variety of commercial products. Experiment with your own mouthwashes; simply blend 1 or 2 drops of peppermint essential oil with 1 cup of vodka or distilled water. Swish with about 2 teaspoons at a time, and then spit it out.

HEALING PROPERTIES

Analgesic
Anti-inflammatory
Antiseptic
Antispasmodic
Astringent
Carminative
Cephalic
Cordial
Decongestant
Emmenagogue
Expectorant
Febrifuge
Stimulant
Sudorific
Vasoconstrictor
Vermifuge

IDEAL FOR TREATING

Cold and flu symptoms
Exhaustion
Hangover
Headaches
Indigestion
Insect bites and bee stings
Itching
Nausea
Rashes
Sunburn
Skin inflammation

Roman Chamomile

ANTHEMIS NOBILIS

BLENDS WELL WITH

Bergamot
Clary sage
Eucalyptus
Frankincense
Geranium
Grapefruit
Helichrysum
Hops
Lavender
Lemon
Lemongrass
Mandarin
Patchouli
Peppermint
Rose
Spearmint
Tea tree
Thyme
Vetiver
Ylang-ylang

SUBSTITUTE WITH

German chamomile
Lavender

Roman chamomile isn't cheap, but it's such a versatile, useful oil that it's worth adding to any small collection. Its pleasant fragrance is floral with fruity, herbal notes that might remind you of the sweet scent of a fresh-picked apple. It can soothe body and mind alike, and is among a handful of essential oils that are safe for infants.

Precautions

◌ Despite Roman chamomile's widespread usefulness in blends that heal skin ailments, it may cause skin irritation in some individuals.

◌ **Do not use during pregnancy.**

◌ May cause allergic reactions in people who are allergic to plants in the daisy family.

◌ Can cause drowsiness. Know how Roman chamomile affects you; if you're among the many who find it very relaxing, do not use it before driving, or while operating machinery.

Application Methods

INHALATION: Blended with 1 cup of steaming water and inhaled, 2 or 3 drops of Roman chamomile can promote a sense of calm. If adding it to a diffuser, use the number of drops recommended by the diffuser's manufacturer.

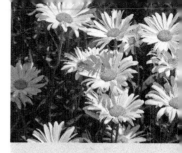

TOPICAL: Blend 2 drops of Roman chamomile essential oil with 4 to 6 drops of carrier oil and rub the mixture onto the soles of your feet at bedtime. You'll enjoy a sense of peaceful relaxation as you drift off to sleep.

BATH: Whether you're in the mood for relaxation or if you're suffering from irritability or PMS symptoms, adding a few drops of Roman chamomile essential oil to your bath water can work wonders. If bloating is a problem, mix up a quick batch of bath salts with 10 drops of Roman chamomile essential oil and 2 cups of Epsom salts. Soak for at least 20 minutes and you'll emerge feeling a bit more like yourself.

Popular Uses

- Keep your skin smooth and healthy with the help of Roman chamomile essential oil. You can create your own daily facial moisturizer, or simply blend a drop of essential oil into a dab of your current moisturizer each time you use it.

- Roman chamomile's soothing scent promotes peaceful sleep, making it a good choice for bedtime baths. Just add 4 to 6 drops to your bathwater and soak for at least 15 minutes.

- Calm children by diffusing Roman chamomile essential oil in the areas where they spend time. Note: This is best for times when relaxation is the goal.

HEALING PROPERTIES
Analgesic
Antibiotic
Antidepressant
Anti-inflammatory
Antiseptic
Antispasmodic
Bactericidal
Carminative
Cholagogue
Cicatrizant
Digestive
Emmenagogue
Febrifuge
Hepatic
Nervine
Sedative
Stomachic
Tonic
Vulnerary

IDEAL FOR TREATING
Diaper rash
Earache
Eczema
Heartburn
Indigestion
Infant teething
Insomnia
Nausea
Stress

Rosemary

ROSMARINUS OFFICINALIS

BLENDS WELL WITH
Basil
Bay laurel
Bergamot
Black pepper
Cedarwood
Clary sage
Clove
Frankincense
Geranium
Grapefruit
Lavender
Lemon
Lemongrass
Mandarin
Niaouli
Oregano
Peppermint
Pine
Tea tree
Thyme

SUBSTITUTE WITH
Basil
Cajeput
Oregano
Peppermint
Thyme

Rosemary is an exceptionally versatile essential oil, with uses that range from soothing cold and flu symptoms, to easing aches and pains. It shines as an addition to hair care products, where it can help dandruff and scalp itch. If you're concerned about hair loss, rosemary essential oil is a must-have: A study published in *Archives of Dermatology* showed that a daily scalp massage with rosemary, thyme, lavender, and cedarwood essential oils blended with carrier oils resulted in 44 percent of patients showing improvement.

Precautions

- **Do not use during pregnancy.**

- Rosemary is a powerful stimulant. It can keep you feeling alert for 3 to 4 hours, so avoid using it within a few hours of your usual bedtime.

- Do not use rosemary if you suffer from epilepsy.

Application Methods

INHALATION: Added to an essential oil inhaler or aromatherapy jewelry, 3 or 4 drops of rosemary essential oil can help you feel alert and focused when studying, driving, or doing creative work. If adding it to a diffuser, use

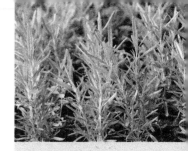

the number of drops recommended by the diffuser's manufacturer.

TOPICAL: Working out? Add 6 drops of rosemary essential oil to 1 teaspoon of your favorite carrier oil for a relaxing massage that soothes stiff, sore muscles.

BATH: Rosemary is a classic ingredient in natural shampoos and conditioners. Try blending it with peppermint, lavender, or lemon for a refreshing aromatherapy delight that doubles as a nourishing treatment for your scalp and hair.

Popular Uses

- Create an ultra-soothing blend for aches and pains by blending rosemary essential oil with equal amounts of peppermint, thyme, and lavender for deep, penetrating comfort. A little goes a long way; dilute with at least an equal amount of carrier oil.

- When work or study gets intense and you really need to focus, blend 20 drops of rosemary essential oil with 40 drops of carrier oil. Keep this blend in a roller bottle and dab it on your temples and pulse points before putting your mind to work.

- If you come down with a cold and need relief from congestion or a sore throat, let rosemary essential oil come to the rescue. It's a potent antiseptic, plus its fragrance helps open up stuffy sinuses.

HEALING PROPERTIES

Analgesic
Antibacterial
Antidepressant
Antifungal
Antimicrobial
Antioxidant
Antiseptic
Antispasmodic
Astringent
Carminative
Cicatrizant
Digestive
Diuretic
Emmenagogue
Hepatic
Hypertensive
Stimulant
Sudorific
Vulnerary

IDEAL FOR TREATING

Bronchitis
Cold and flu
  symptoms
Dandruff
Fatigue
Indigestion
Nervousness
Sinusitis
Thinning hair
Varicose veins

Tea Tree

MELALEUCA ALTERNIFOLIA

BLENDS WELL WITH

Basil
Bergamot
Black pepper
Cinnamon
Clary sage
Clove
Cypress
Eucalyptus
Geranium
Juniper
Lavender
Lemon
Lime
Myrrh
Orange
Oregano
Peppermint
Rosemary
Spearmint
Thyme

SUBSTITUTE WITH

Clove
Eucalyptus
Lavender

Sometimes referred to simply as mela-leuca, tea tree essential oil is effective for dealing with fungus, treating minor wounds, and clearing up a variety of minor infections. In a 2013 study published by the *International Journal of Dermatology*, tea tree essential oil was shown to exhibit high levels of antimicrobial and anti-inflammatory action, with effective-ness against bacteria, viruses, fungi, and protozoal infections. Among its proven uses are treating acne, seborrheic derma-titis, and gingivitis. Tea tree essential oil has also been proven to help wounds heal faster, so add it to your natural first-aid kit.

Precautions

- Generally regarded as safe.

Application Methods

INHALATION: Mixed into 1 cup of steaming hot water, a few drops of tea tree essential oil can soothe respiratory discomfort. If adding to a diffuser, use the number of drops recom-mended by the diffuser's manufacturer.

TOPICAL: Tea tree essential oil can be used neat on minor cuts and scrapes. Just drip a drop onto the affected area and allow it to air-dry.

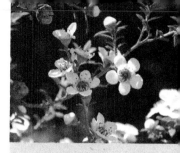

BATH: If you have dandruff, try adding tea tree essential oil to your shampoo. It kills fungus and helps your scalp heal, while cutting down on itchiness.

Popular Uses

- During cold and flu season, add tea tree essential oil to a vaporizer for relief from congestion.

- Tea tree essential oil helps sunburns heal faster. Blend it with aloe vera gel on its own or with complementary essential oils, and apply it liberally to affected areas a few times each day until the skin heals.

- Tea tree's powerful antiviral, antifungal, and antibacterial qualities make it an excellent addition to household cleaners. Used on its own or blended with other essential oils, tea tree essential oil keeps a variety of surfaces fresh and clean.

HEALING PROPERTIES

Antimicrobial
Antiseptic
Antiviral
Bactericide
Cicatrizant
Expectorant
Fungicide
Insecticide
Insect repellent
Stimulant
Sudorific

IDEAL FOR TREATING

Acne
Athlete's foot
Body odor
Cold and flu care
Dandruff
Gingivitis
Insect bites and
  bee stings
Insect infestation
Jock itch
Minor burns
Minor cuts
  and scrapes
Nail fungus
Oily skin and hair
Ringworm
Swimmer's ear
Yeast infection

Thyme

THYMUS VULGARIS

Thyme's fresh, herbal scent provides quite an energy boost when you're feeling drained. This wonderful essential oil offers a variety of benefits: Use it to balance and heal skin or ease PMS and menopause symptoms. Thyme's expectorant property can help alleviate upper respiratory symptoms associated with colds and flu, while its antifungal constituents are ideal for treating athlete's foot, ringworm, jock itch, and nail fungus.

Precautions

- Thyme is a "hot" essential oil that needs to be carefully diluted before use.

- If you are sensitive to peppermint or rosemary essential oil, you will likely find thyme equally irritating.

- **Do not use during pregnancy.**

- Do not use topically on children under age 6 years.

- Thyme can stimulate the thyroid gland and should be avoided by those with hyperthyroidism.

- Because thyme can raise blood pressure, it is not suitable for use with those who have elevated blood pressure.

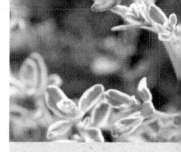

Application Methods

INHALATION: Mixed into 1 cup of steaming hot water, a few drops of thyme essential oil provide quick relief from cold and flu symptoms. If adding thyme to a diffuser, use the number of drops recommended by the diffuser's manufacturer.

TOPICAL: Blend 3 to 4 drops of thyme essential oil with 1 teaspoon of carrier oil and apply it to the chest area for relief from congestion.

BATH: Adding a few drops of thyme essential oil to your bathwater can help you de-stress and ease anxiety.

Popular Uses

- For acne and other irritations, dilute thyme essential oil with an equal amount of carrier oil and apply once or twice daily until skin clears.

- Thyme's ability to boost energy makes it ideal for adding to diffuser blends that promote clarity and focus. Try it with rosemary, peppermint or spearmint, lemon or lemongrass, or any combination of oils that prompt alertness.

- Thanks to its ability to relieve joint and muscle pain, thyme is an outstanding addition to hot and cold compresses as well as balms, salves, and massage oils.

HEALING PROPERTIES

Antibacterial
Antifungal
Antimicrobial
Antioxidant
Antiseptic
Antispasmodic
Antitussive
Astringent
Cicatrizant
Disinfectant
Expectorant
Hypertensive
Insecticide
Insect repellent
Stimulant
Sudorific

IDEAL FOR TREATING

Aging skin
Anxiety
Cold and flu symptoms
Diarrhea
Fatigue
Hair loss
Hangover
Nervousness
PMS
Stress
Upper respiratory infections

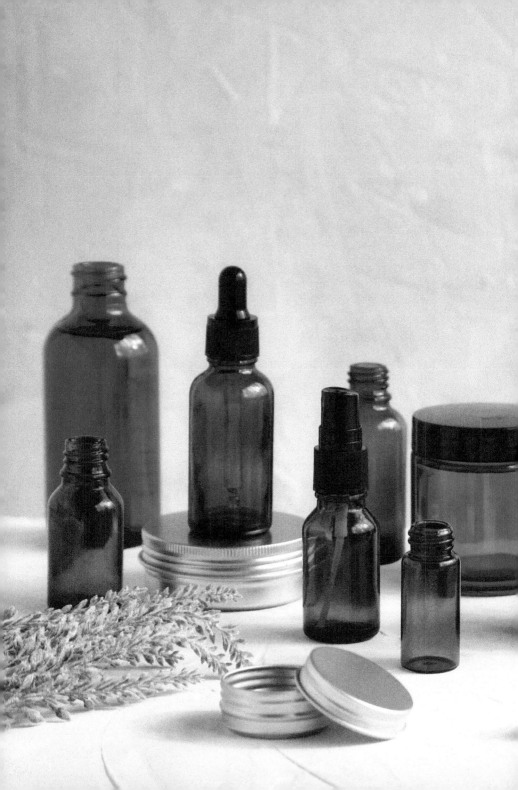

PART TWO

Remedies, Recipes, & Applications

Aromatherapy can be used for a wide variety of ailments, and essential oils offer countless emotional benefits.

Some remedies call for a single essential oil, while others recreate popular commercial synergy blends. The "Must Have" recipe label indicates remedies that can be made with any of the nine "must have" essential oils: clove, eucalyptus, geranium, lavender, lemon, lemongrass, peppermint, rosemary, and tea tree. Additional recipe labels include the following:

Aromatic: Benefits come from inhalation.

May Cause Photosensitivity: The essential oils in this recipe may increase sensitivity to the sun, leading to sunburn. Most literature advises users to protect treated areas from the sun for 12 to 24 hours after use.

Safe for Ages 2+, 6+ 12+, or All Ages: This icon indicates the safe age range for users based on topically applied essential oils, and/or the concentration level in the remedy.

Topical: Benefits come from application to the skin.

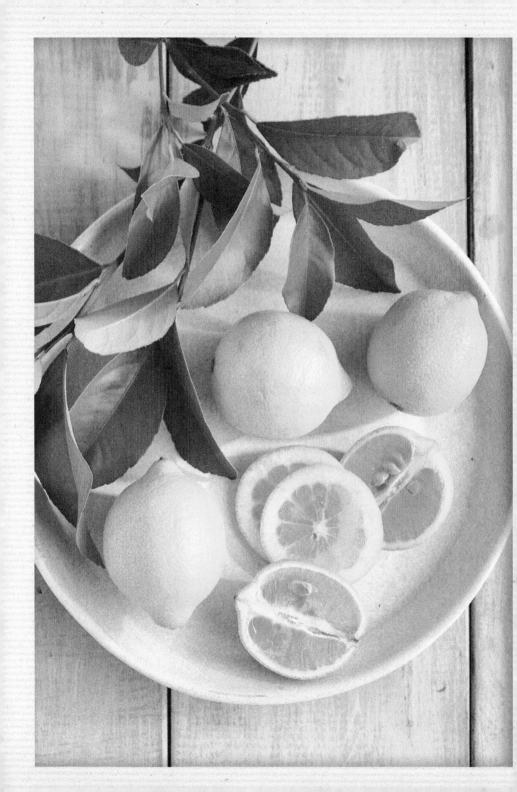

CHAPTER 5

Remedies for Everyday Health and Ailments

Since ancient times, people from all walks of life have used essential oils to improve their well-being. In this chapter, you'll find 35 of the most commonly treated ailments, plus simple ways to harness the healing power of aromatherapy to address them.

Allergies

Seasonal sniffling, sneezing, and congestion make for miserable warm-weather outings. When you have allergies, your immune system works overtime, trying to eliminate irritants it views as threats. Aromatherapy provides natural relief, without the side effects that can accompany conventional medications. Simply diffusing essential oils or adding them to aromatherapy inhalers can help.

Note: If you're allergic to ragweed, don't use Roman chamomile; it will make your symptoms worse.

Helpful Essential Oils: clove, eucalyptus, lavender, lemon, peppermint, Roman chamomile (see Note), rosemary

PEPPERMINT-EUCALYPTUS VAPOR RUB

AROMATIC, TOPICAL, SAFE FOR CHILDREN AGES 6+

MUST HAVE   Peppermint essential oil contains menthol, which reduces respiratory inflammation. It also has anticongestive effects, helping you breathe better. Eucalyptus essential oil offers similar benefits, and rounds out the sharp scent of peppermint. This vapor rub isn't just for allergy season; make a batch to help ease the sniffles that accompany colds and flu. MAKES ABOUT ½ CUP

20 drops eucalyptus essential oil
25 drops peppermint essential oil
¼ cup coconut oil, at room
    temperature

¼ cup mango butter, at room
    temperature

1. In a medium bowl, combine the eucalyptus and peppermint essential oils.

2. Add the coconut oil and mango butter (see Tip). With an electric mixer, whip the ingredients until completely combined. Transfer the blend to a clean, dry jar with a tight-fitting lid.

3. With your fingertips, apply just enough vapor rub to cover the upper chest with a thin layer. Repeat as needed throughout the day.

4. Store your rub in a cool, dark place between uses.

Tip: If you're missing one of the essential oils in the recipe, use just one oil or create a new blend with any of the recommended allergy-fighting oils. Similarly, if you don't have mango butter, use coconut or shea butter.

AROMATIC, SAFE FOR CHILDREN AGES 2+

Let aromatherapy come to the rescue when allergies make it hard to relax and fall asleep. This blend smells lovely, and helps keep your airways clear, while promoting a sense of calm. You can easily multiply this recipe to make a larger batch to keep on hand.

MAKES ABOUT 20 TREATMENTS

25 drops eucalyptus essential oil
20 drops lavender essential oil
10 drops lemon essential oil
25 drops peppermint essential oil

10 drops Roman chamomile
essential oil
5 drops tea tree essential oil

1. In a dark-colored glass bottle, combine the eucalyptus, lavender, lemon, peppermint, Roman chamomile, and tea tree essential oils. Let the blend rest for at least 1 hour before use.

2. Add 3 to 5 drops of the finished blend to a diffuser and use according to the manufacturer's instructions.

3. Store the blend in a cool place between uses.

Tip: This blend isn't just for diffusing: It's also ideal for use in an aromatherapy inhaler or aromatherapy jewelry, or add a few drops to a warm bath.

Asthma

While essential oils are not suitable for use during an asthma attack, you may be able to reduce your symptoms with aromatherapy, especially if your case is mild. Never discontinue prescription medications without your doctor's consent.

Helpful Essential Oils: clary sage, eucalyptus, frankincense, geranium, lavender, lemon, peppermint, Roman chamomile, thyme

CLARY SAGE MASSAGE

TOPICAL, SAFE FOR CHILDREN 12+

Clary sage offers strong antispasmodic action, and its ability to relax tight muscles and ease anxiety can help fight asthma. This recipe uses jojoba oil, which has a very light feel and absorbs rapidly. While nice to have, jojoba isn't essential; use whatever carrier oil you have on hand. MAKES ABOUT 2 TABLESPOONS

2 tablespoons jojoba oil   30 drops clary sage essential oil

1. In a glass bottle with a tight-fitting lid, combine the jojoba oil and clary sage essential oil. Cover and shake well to blend.

2. Apply 5 to 7 drops of massage oil to your chest and neck, inhaling deeply. Repeat as needed.

3. Store the massage oil in a cool, dark place between uses.

Tip: If you have no clary sage on hand, try this massage with another anti-asthma oil.

LAVENDER-ROMAN CHAMOMILE STEAM

AROMATIC, SAFE FOR CHILDREN AGES 6+

Lavender and Roman chamomile essential oils help tight, constricted airways relax and offers relief from anxiety, while the steam eases congestive discomfort. This blend is ideal for anyone who suffers from frequent asthma attacks, and it provides soothing relief after attacks end. If you like, use an aromatherapy inhaler, aromatherapy jewelry, or a diffuser. MAKES 1 TREATMENT

2 cups steaming hot water   3 drops Roman chamomile
   (not boiling)   essential oil
8 drops lavender essential oil

1. In a large shallow bowl, combine the hot water with the lavender and Roman chamomile essential oils.

2. Place the bowl on a towel-topped table, and sit comfortably in front of the bowl.

3. Breathe slowly and deeply over the bowl until the water cools. Repeat as needed.

Tip: While this strong steam treatment isn't suitable for children under age 6 years, you can treat them to a safe aromatherapy experience by placing the essential oils in a warm bath and allowing them to soak for at least 10 minutes.

Athlete's Foot

You don't have to be a dedicated gym-goer to suffer from athlete's foot; this itchy, painful fungal infection can happen to anyone. Keep your feet clean and dry while recovering, and expose them to fresh air as often as you can.

Helpful Essential Oils: clove, lavender, lemon, lemongrass, patchouli, rosemary, tea tree, thyme

TEA TREE FOOT POWDER

TOPICAL, SAFE FOR CHILDREN AGES 6+

MUST HAVE Tea tree essential oil's powerful antifungal action makes it one of the best natural athlete's foot remedies available. This powder can help you heal around the clock, even when you can't treat your feet to a soak or expose them to fresh air. MAKES 1 CUP

1 cup baby powder, preferably talc- and fragrance-free

40 drops tea tree essential oil

1. In a sugar shaker, add the baby powder.

2. Using a thin utensil, such as a fork or butter knife, stir in the tea tree essential oil, about 5 drops at a time.

3. Once combined, cap tightly, cover the holes in the lid, and shake well to ensure thorough blending.

4. After bathing or showering, dry your feet well, focusing on the areas between your toes. Apply a generous dusting of foot powder, covering all affected areas. Repeat as needed, at least twice daily.

5. Keep your foot powder in a cool, dark, dry place between uses.

   Tip: Use this powder to disinfect and deodorize shoes after wearing them.

ANTIFUNGAL FOOT BALM

TOPICAL, SAFE FOR CHILDREN AGES 12+

MUST HAVE In this soothing balm, tea tree, lemongrass, and lavender essential oils combine with coconut oil, which also offers antifungal properties. Don't be surprised if you find yourself using this remedy after your case of athlete's foot clears up! It smells wonderful and it helps keep your feet feeling soft.

MAKES ABOUT ½ CUP

20 drops lavender essential oil

40 drops lemongrass essential oil

20 drops tea tree essential oil

½ cup coconut oil, barely melted

1. In a glass jar with a tight-fitting lid, combine the lavender, lemongrass, and tea tree essential oils.

2. Using a thin utensil, such as a fork or butter knife, stir in the coconut oil to blend.

3. After bathing or showering, dry your feet well, focusing on the areas between your toes. Apply a thin layer of foot balm and allow it to absorb before walking.

4. Keep your foot balm in a cool, dark place between uses.

   Tip: Indulge in a soothing, extra-moisturizing treatment by coating your feet with a heavier layer of foot balm and putting on your most comfortable pair of socks. Wear the socks for at least 1 hour, or even overnight. When you take the socks off, your feet will feel fantastic.

Blisters

Although they are small, blisters can be quite painful! Resist the urge to pop them, since the liquid inside provides a cushion and helps your blister heal faster. Essential oils can provide some welcome relief from the discomfort and prevent infection both before and after your blister deflates on its own.

Helpful Essential Oils: eucalyptus, frankincense, geranium, lavender, lemon, peppermint, Roman chamomile, tea tree

LAVENDER NEAT TREATMENT

TOPICAL, SAFE FOR CHILDREN AGES 6+

MUST HAVE Lavender offers pain relief and helps prevent blisters from becoming infected. With consistent use, it may even help your blister disappear faster. You can use this treatment on a blister before it pops, and you'll find it is particularly soothing if the blister pops or tears open. MAKES 1 TREATMENT

1 drop lavender essential oil

1. Drip a single drop of lavender essential oil onto the blister. Repeat 2 to 3 times daily until the blister heals.

2. If the blister pops, cover the treated area with an adhesive bandage to prevent further injury.

   Tip: If a child under 6 years has a blister, you can treat it with lavender. Mix 8 drops lavender essential oil with 1 tablespoon coconut oil and apply the remedy 1 drop at a time. Keep the blend in a sealed container in a cool, dark place between uses.

SYNERGISTIC BLISTER BALM

TOPICAL, MAY CAUSE PHOTOSENSITIVITY, SAFE FOR CHILDREN AGES 12+

Lavender, tea tree, and Roman chamomile essential oils pair with soothing coconut oil to reduce pain and promote faster healing. If you're treating an unbroken blister, add peppermint essential oil to the blend for added pain relief. MAKES ABOUT 2 TABLESPOONS

40 drops lavender essential oil

20 drops Roman chamomile essential oil

5 drops tea tree essential oil

5 drops peppermint essential oil (optional)

2 tablespoons coconut oil, barely melted

1. In a glass jar with a tight-fitting lid, combine the lavender, Roman chamomile, tea tree, and peppermint (if using) essential oils. Let the blend rest for at least 1 hour.

2. Using a thin utensil, such as a fork or butter knife, stir in the coconut oil until well blended.

3. With clean fingertips or a cotton swab, apply a pea-size amount of balm to each blister. Repeat 2 to 3 times daily until the blister heals.

4. If the blister pops, cover the treated area with an adhesive bandage to prevent further injury.

5. Keep your blister balm in a cool, dark place between uses.

Tip: Missing an oil or two? You can still create a synergistic blend with any of the oils in this recipe, or others from the list of blister-healing essential oils.

Bronchitis

Bronchitis may be caused by a viral infection, exposure to lung irritants, or a bacterial infection. Aromatherapy can help with the discomfort and inflammation, and the antibacterial and antiviral properties of the essential oils may help reduce infection. Chronic bronchitis can lead to pneumonia, so it's important to check with your doctor to be sure aromatherapy isn't contraindicated for use alongside prescribed medication.

Helpful Essential Oils: clove, eucalyptus, frankincense, lavender, lemon, peppermint, rosemary, thyme

FRANKINCENSE-CLOVE MASSAGE

TOPICAL, SAFE FOR CHILDREN AGES 6+

Frankincense and clove essential oils offer antibacterial properties, plus their warm, spicy fragrances soothe inflamed airways. If you don't want to apply a topical remedy, you can enjoy a similar effect by adding the blend to an essential oil inhaler, aromatherapy jewelry, or a diffuser. MAKES ABOUT ¼ CUP

5 drops clove essential oil
20 drops frankincense
    essential oil

¼ cup jojoba oil

1. In a glass bottle or jar with a tight-fitting lid, combine the clove and frankincense essential oils. Let the blend rest for at least 1 hour.

2. Add the jojoba oil, cover the container, and shake well to combine.

3. With your fingertips, apply 4 to 6 drops of the blend to the chest and throat area. Repeat as needed throughout the day.

4. Keep the massage oil in a cool, dark place between uses.

Tip: For children under 6 years, double the dilution rate by using half the amount of each essential oil.

ROSEMARY BRONCHITIS STEAM

AROMATIC, SAFE FOR CHILDREN AGES 6+

MUST HAVE Rosemary essential oil and steam provide soothing relief from uncomfortable bronchitis symptoms. You can add 1 drop of peppermint, 1 drop of lemon, and/or 1 drop of eucalyptus essential oils to this treatment for a stronger effect.

MAKES 1 TREATMENT

2 cups steaming hot water (not boiling)	3 drops rosemary essential oil

1. In a large shallow bowl, combine the hot water and rosemary essential oil.

2. Place the bowl on a towel-topped table, and sit comfortably in front of the bowl.

3. Breathe slowly and deeply over the bowl until the water cools. Repeat as needed.

Tip: While this strong steam treatment isn't suitable for children under 6 years, you can treat them to a safe aromatherapy experience by placing the essential oil in a warm bath and allowing them to soak for at least 10 minutes.

Bruises

Next time you stumble in the dark and bark your shin, treat your bruises to some much-needed TLC. Essential oils ease the pain that accompanies bruising, plus they help compromised tissues heal faster. If you don't have the oils needed to create a synergistic blend, try applying 1 drop of lavender essential oil mixed with 1 drop of carrier oil. It might just do the trick.

Helpful Essential Oils: clove, frankincense, geranium, lavender, lemon, Roman chamomile, rosemary, tea tree

SYNERGISTIC BRUISE BALM

TOPICAL, MAY CAUSE PHOTOSENSITIVITY, SAFE FOR CHILDREN AGES 6+

MUST HAVE Lavender, lemon, rosemary, and tea tree essential oils have anti-inflammatory effects, and help increase circulation so tissues heal faster. They can also take some of the sting out of painful bruises. MAKES ABOUT 2 TABLESPOONS

40 drops lavender essential oil
20 drops lemon essential oil
5 drops rosemary essential oil

5 drops tea tree essential oil
2 tablespoons coconut oil, barely melted

1. In a glass jar with a tight-fitting lid, combine the lavender, lemon, rosemary, and tea tree essential oils. Let the blend rest for at least 1 hour.

2. Using a thin utensil, such as a fork or butter knife, stir in the coconut oil until well blended.

3. With clean fingertips or a cotton pad, apply a pea-sized amount of balm to each bruise, using a little more or less as needed. Repeat 2 to 3 times daily until bruises fade.

4. Keep your bruise balm in a cool, dark place between uses.

Tip: Missing an oil or two? You can still create a synergistic blend with any of the oils in this recipe and others from the list of blister-healing essential oils.

LAVENDER-CLOVE COMPRESS

AROMATIC, SAFE FOR CHILDREN AGES 2+

MUST HAVE If you have a fresh, painful bruise, you can use a combination of a cold compress and essential oils to numb the pain and promote faster healing. If you have no ice pack handy, use a bag of frozen vegetables instead—peas are a fantastic stand-in.

MAKES 1 TREATMENT

1 drop clove essential oil   3 drops olive oil
2 drops lavender essential oil

1. In a small dish or cup, mix the clove and lavender essential oils with the olive oil.

2. Using your fingertips or a cotton pad, apply the entire amount to your bruise and the surrounding area.

3. Wrap an ice pack in a soft cloth and apply it to the bruise. Leave it in place for at least 5 minutes. Repeat as needed.

Tip: You can combine 1 drop lavender essential oil with 10 drops olive oil to treat bruises on children younger than 2 years. The blend will help even if your child cannot tolerate the cold of an ice pack.

Burns

Aromatherapy is suitable for treating minor burns; with essential oils, you can ease the pain, reduce the likelihood of infection, and help skin heal faster. With prompt attention, you may even be able to reduce scarring. Keep in mind that severe burns require immediate, professional emergency medical care.

Helpful Essential Oils: eucalyptus, frankincense, lavender, peppermint, tea tree

LAVENDER BURN GEL

TOPICAL, SAFE FOR ALL AGES

MUST HAVE Aloe vera gel stimulates healing and provides cool comfort to burns, while acting as a carrier for lavender essential oil. Look for a brand with no added color, and keep it refrigerated so it lasts longer. If you have a green thumb, consider growing your own aloe. MAKES ABOUT 2 TABLESPOONS

2 tablespoons aloe vera gel   20 drops lavender essential oil

1. In a small bowl, combine the aloe vera gel and lavender essential oil. With a small whisk or fork, stir until well combined.

2. Transfer the blend to a container with a tight-fitting lid. A plastic squeeze-type travel bottle is ideal.

3. With clean fingertips or a cotton pad, apply a pea-sized amount of gel to the burn. Don't worry about rubbing it in; even a thick layer will absorb eventually. Let the area air-dry and repeat as needed until the burn heals.

4. Keep the gel refrigerated between uses.

   Tip: If you don't have aloe vera gel, use coconut oil or another carrier.

LAVENDER-FRANKINCENSE BURN BALM

TOPICAL, SAFE FOR ALL AGES

Lavender and frankincense essential oils, vitamin E, and coconut oil team up to repair skin faster. Besides offering a soothing, healing influence, frankincense and lavender can help prevent or minimize scar formation, particularly if you keep applying them until the burn is completely healed. MAKES ABOUT 2 TABLESPOONS

20 drops frankincense essential oil	2 vitamin E capsules
15 drops lavender essential oil	2 tablespoons coconut oil, barely melted

1. In a glass jar with a tight-fitting lid, combine the frankincense and lavender essential oils. If you have time, let them rest for at least 1 hour before continuing.

2. With sharp scissors, carefully snip a small hole in each vitamin E capsule, and squeeze the contents into the jar with the essential oils.

3. Using a thin utensil, such as a fork or butter knife, stir in the coconut oil until well combined.

4. With your fingertips or a cotton swab, gently apply a pea-sized amount of balm to the burned area, using a little more or less as needed. Repeat 2 to 3 times daily.

5. Keep the balm in a cool, dark place between uses.

Tip: If you're preparing this remedy for adults or children over age 2 years, you can add 5 drops of tea tree essential oil and/ or 5 drops of peppermint essential oil to the blend for added pain relief.

AROMATHERAPY FOR BEGINNERS

Chicken Pox

While the varicella vaccine has reduced the number of chicken pox cases, it's still a common and contagious virus. Antiviral essential oils can help make you or your child more comfortable, and may even reduce the severity and number of pox blisters. If possible, consider making both blends and using them one after another for stronger relief.

Helpful Essential Oils: eucalyptus, frankincense, lavender, Roman chamomile, tea tree

HEALING BATH

TOPICAL, SAFE FOR CHILDREN AGES 6+

MUST HAVE Eucalyptus and tea tree essential oils offer strong antiviral action, while helping prevent infection. The lukewarm water will help your little one feel more comfortable and it's fine for him to stay in the bathtub for longer than the recommended minimum 10 minutes. MAKES 1 TREATMENT

2 drops eucalyptus essential oil   2 drops tea tree essential oil

1. Fill a bathtub with lukewarm water. Use the same amount you normally do for your child's bath.

2. Add the essential oils to the water and place your child in the tub. Encourage your child to play with toys, or read him a story, to keep him in the tub for at least 10 minutes.

3. After bathing, pat your child dry with a soft towel.

   Tip: If your child is under 6 years, you can create a soothing bath with tea tree essential oil and a milder essential oil. Substitute 2 drops of lavender, Roman chamomile, or frankincense essential oil for the eucalyptus.

ANTI-ITCH SPRAY

TOPICAL, SAFE FOR ALL AGES

Witch hazel is a well-known remedy for cooling itchy chicken pox, easing inflammation. Together with soothing essential oils that promote healing and have a calming influence, your child will feel more comfortable. MAKES ABOUT ½ CUP

10 drops lavender essential oil

10 drops frankincense
essential oil

10 drops Roman chamomile
essential oil

¼ cup alcohol-free witch hazel

3½ tablespoons water

1½ teaspoons aloe vera gel

1. In a bottle fitted with a spray top, combine the lavender, frankincense, and Roman chamomile essential oils. Let them rest for at least 1 hour before continuing.

2. Add the witch hazel, water, and aloe vera gel, cover the container, and shake well to combine.

3. Shake the bottle again before each use. Gently spritz each affected area and allow it to air-dry. For chicken pox on the face, or for children who don't respond well to spraying, use cotton pads to gently swab on the treatment. Repeat as needed throughout the day.

4. Keep the spray refrigerated between uses.

Tip: You can make a similar spray even if you don't have all the recommended ingredients. Simply increase the amount of the essential oils you do have to equal 30 drops; for example, use 15 drops of lavender essential oil and 15 drops of Roman chamomile essential oil.

Cold and Flu Care

Cold and flu symptoms such as sore throat, coughing, sneezing, and congestion call for plenty of TLC. Besides offering comfort, treatments that include antibacterial, antiviral, and antiseptic essential oils can help you get over your symptoms faster. You can try these on their own or use them alongside other remedies. If you're on antibiotics, ask your doctor if it's okay to use aromatherapy for symptom management.

Helpful Essential Oils: clove, eucalyptus, frankincense, lemon, peppermint, Roman chamomile, rosemary, tea tree, thyme

COMFORTING EUCALYPTUS STEAM

AROMATIC, SAFE FOR CHILDREN AGES 6+

MUST HAVE · Eucalyptus and steam combine to clear congestion, loosen phlegm, and help you feel more comfortable. If you have a sore throat, add 1 drop of peppermint and/or 1 drop of rosemary or thyme essential oil to this treatment for a stronger effect.

MAKES 1 TREATMENT

2 cups steaming hot water (not boiling)

4 drops eucalyptus essential oil

1. In a large, shallow bowl, combine the hot water and eucalyptus essential oil.

2. Place the bowl on a towel-topped table, and sit comfortably in front of the bowl.

3. Breathe slowly and deeply until the water cools. Repeat as needed.

Tip: While this strong steam treatment isn't suitable for children under 6 years, you can treat them to a safe aromatherapy experience by placing 2 drops eucalyptus essential oil in a warm bath and allowing them to soak for at least 10 minutes.

ROSEMARY-LEMON GARGLE

TOPICAL, SAFE FOR CHILDREN AGES 12+

MUST HAVE Essential oils can soothe sore throats quickly, killing bacteria at the same time. If treating a child, be sure he or she knows how to gargle safely, without swallowing any of the water. It won't hurt if a little is swallowed accidentally, but ingesting essential oils is best practiced under the supervision of a knowledgeable practitioner. MAKES 1 TREATMENT

½ cup lukewarm water
3 drops lemon essential oil

1 drop rosemary essential oil

1. In a cup, combine the water with the lemon and rosemary essential oils.

2. Gargle with a small amount and then spit it out into the sink. Repeat until the entire amount has been used.

3. Repeat 2 to 3 times throughout the day.

Tip: Severe sore throats sometimes call for something stronger. If this remedy isn't working, try replacing the rosemary essential oil with 1 drop of clove essential oil.

DECONGESTANT VAPOR RUB

TOPICAL, MAY CAUSE PHOTOSENSITIVITY, SAFE FOR CHILDREN AGES 6+

Antiseptic, antibacterial, and immune-stimulating essential oils come together in this vapor rub, which feels far less greasy than the commercial kind. This remedy is just the thing for stuffy noses, sore throats, and troublesome coughs. Note: This rub isn't as strong-smelling as commercial variants. If you need something stronger for a person older than age 6 years, double the amount of each essential oil used. MAKES ABOUT 1 CUP

2 drops clove essential oil
10 drops eucalyptus essential oil
10 drops lemon essential oil
5 drops rosemary essential oil
10 drops tea tree essential oil

5 drops thyme essential oil
½ cup coconut oil, at room temperature
½ cup mango butter, at room temperature (see Tip)

1. In a small bowl, combine the clove, eucalyptus, lemon, rosemary, tea tree, and thyme essential oils.

2. Add the coconut oil and the mango butter. With an electric mixer, whip the ingredients until they are completely combined. Transfer the blend to a clean, dry jar with a tight-fitting lid.

3. With your fingertips, apply just enough vapor rub to cover the upper chest with a thin layer. Repeat as needed throughout the day.

Tip: If you're missing any of the essential oils in the recipe, you can use just one oil or create a new blend with any of the recommended cold- and flu-fighting oils. If mango butter is not available, use shea or coconut butter.

Cuts and Scrapes

Kitchen accidents, playground boo-boos, and owies of all kinds respond well to treatment with essential oils. Aromatherapy is reserved for minor injuries. There are many stories about how major injuries were successfully treated with essential oils, and they can often be used alongside conventional treatment, but always seek emergency medical treatment for any major injury.

Helpful Essential Oils: clove, eucalyptus, lavender, frankincense, Roman chamomile, tea tree

A DASH OF LAVENDER

TOPICAL, SAFE FOR CHILDREN AGES 6+

MUST HAVE Lavender essential oil speeds healing, acts as a natural antibacterial agent, and takes some of the sting out of minor injuries of all kinds. This treatment is super simple and it's a favorite with many who use aromatherapy. MAKES 1 TREATMENT

1 drop lavender essential oil

1. Wash the affected area and allow it to air-dry.

2. Apply 1 drop of lavender essential oil with an eyedropper, or straight from the bottle. Allow the oil to air-dry. Cover the injury with an adhesive bandage, if needed. Repeat once or twice daily until healed.

Tip: If a child under 6 years has a minor cut or scrape, you can treat it with lavender. Mix 10 drops lavender essential oil with 1 tablespoon coconut oil and apply the remedy 1 drop at a time. Keep the blend in a sealed container in a cool, dark place between uses.

ROMAN CHAMOMILE, CLOVE, AND TEA TREE BALM

TOPICAL, SAFE FOR CHILDREN 6+

Clove, Roman chamomile, and tea tree essential oils combine with aloe vera gel to soothe minor wounds and help them heal faster. Look for clear aloe vera gel; it's available at most drugstores and some supermarkets. MAKES ABOUT 2 TABLESPOONS

2 drops clove essential oil

20 drops Roman chamomile essential oil

10 drops tea tree essential oil

2 tablespoons aloe vera gel

1. In a small bowl, combine the clove, Roman chamomile, and tea tree essential oils with the aloe vera gel. Using a small whisk or fork, blend until well combined. Transfer the blend to a container with a tight-fitting lid. A plastic squeeze-type travel bottle is ideal for this remedy.

2. With clean fingertips or a cotton pad, apply a pea-size amount of gel to the cut or scrape, using a little more or less as needed. Don't worry about applying too much or rubbing it in; even a thick layer will absorb eventually. Let the area air-dry and repeat as needed until the wound heals.

3. Store the gel in the refrigerator between uses.

   Tip: If you don't have aloe gel, use coconut oil in its place.

Cramped or Painful Muscles

Whether you've overdone it at the gym, spent long hours working, or suffered a minor injury—aromatherapy offers quick relief for painful muscles. However, if you have a serious injury or suspect you've hurt your neck or back, seek prompt medical attention. You may be able to continue using essential oils for natural pain relief, as long as your doctor gives consent.

Helpful Essential Oils: clary sage, clove, eucalyptus, grapefruit, lavender, lemon, lemongrass, peppermint, Roman chamomile

COOLING MUSCLE MASSAGE

TOPICAL, SAFE FOR CHILDREN AGES 6+

Clary sage, lemongrass, and peppermint essential oils penetrate deeply and provide pain relief, while simultaneously calming your mind. If you have no clary sage or lemongrass, try this remedy with peppermint essential oil alone; use 20 drops instead of 10.

MAKES ABOUT ¼ CUP

| 10 drops clary sage essential oil | 10 drops peppermint essential oil |
| 10 drops lemongrass essential oil | ¼ cup jojoba oil |

1. In a glass bottle or jar with a tight-fitting lid, combine the clary sage, lemongrass, and peppermint essential oils. Let them rest for at least 1 hour.

2. Add the jojoba oil, cover the container, and shake well to combine.

3. With your fingertips, apply 4 to 6 drops to the affected area, using a little more or less as needed. Massage using gentle circular motions and repeat as needed throughout the day.

4. Store the massage oil in a cool, dark place between uses.

Tip: Jojoba oil is ideal for massage oil since it absorbs quickly, but any carrier oil will work, even plain olive oil from the kitchen.

LAVENDER-THYME BODY BALM

TOPICAL, SAFE FOR CHILDREN AGES 6+

Soothing lavender and warming thyme essential oils comfort overworked muscles. For a slightly stronger remedy, add 4 drops of peppermint essential oil to this blend. For a more relaxing effect, add 10 drops of clary sage. MAKES ABOUT 1 CUP

30 drops lavender essential oil	½ cup mango butter, or coconut
20 drops thyme essential oil	or shea butter, at room
½ cup coconut oil, at room	temperature
temperature	

1. In a small bowl, combine the lavender and thyme essential oils.

2. Add the coconut oil and mango butter. With an electric mixer, whip the ingredients until completely combined. Transfer the blend to a clean, dry jar with a tight-fitting lid.

3. With your fingertips, apply just enough balm to cover the affected area with a thin layer. Massage using gentle circular motions and repeat as needed.

4. Keep your body balm in a cool, dark place between uses.

   Tip: For a faster remedy with no mixing, replace the coconut oil and mango butter with 1 cup of your favorite carrier oil. Fractionated coconut oil, jojoba oil, and sweet almond oil are some popular ones to try.

Diaper Rash

Diaper rash can occur even when you try your best to prevent it. Like conventional treatments, aromatherapy works best when you tackle symptoms as soon as they appear. If you suspect your baby has an infection, or if the problem gets worse instead of improving, see your pediatrician.

Helpful Essential Oils: frankincense, lavender, Roman chamomile

SOOTHING BUM WASH

TOPICAL, SAFE FOR ALL AGES

Aloe vera and soothing, baby-safe essential oils help cool the sting of diaper rash and promote faster healing. If your little one is over the age of 3 months, you can double the amount of essential oil for a slightly stronger wash. When choosing aloe for baby products, look for an alcohol-free brand with no added color or fragrance.

MAKES ABOUT 1 CUP

2 drops frankincense essential oil

2 drops lavender essential oil

2 drops Roman chamomile
essential oil

2 tablespoons aloe vera gel

¾ cup purified water

1. In a bottle or jar with a tight-fitting lid, combine the frankincense, lavender, and Roman chamomile essential oils. Let them rest for at least 1 hour.

2. Add the aloe vera gel and the purified water. Cap the container and shake it well to combine the ingredients. Give the bottle a shake before each use.

3. After each diaper change, and after using cleansing wipes to sanitize your baby's bottom, moisten a soft cloth or cotton pad with at least 1 teaspoon of bum wash. Gently apply the wash to all affected areas.

4. Let the skin air-dry and use a barrier cream for protection.

5. Keep the wash in a cool, dark place between uses.

Tip: If you like, and if your baby will tolerate it, keep this wash in a spray bottle and spritz it on instead of dabbing.

LAVENDER-FRANKINCENSE CREAM

TOPICAL, SAFE FOR ALL AGES

Lavender and frankincense essential oil join antibacterial coconut oil and natural lanolin to provide a moisture barrier and promote faster healing. If your baby is over 3 months old, you can double the amount of essential oils for a stronger remedy. It's best to choose organic oils whenever possible, and it is particularly important here due to the sensitive nature of the application.

MAKES ABOUT ½ CUP

5 drops frankincense essential oil
3 drops lavender essential oil
2 tablespoons lanolin,
    barely melted

6 tablespoons organic coconut
    oil, barely melted

1. In a shallow bowl, combine the frankincense and lavender essential oils.

2. Add the lanolin and coconut oil. With a clean, dry whisk, blend the ingredients well. Transfer the finished cream to a clean, dry jar with a tight-fitting lid.

3. At each diaper change, use your fingertips or a cotton pad to apply a thin layer of cream to your baby's diaper area after it is completely dry—about ½ teaspoon should be enough.

4. Keep the cream in a cool, dark place between uses.

Tip: If you can't find lanolin, replace it with an equal amount of shea butter, or just make this recipe with ½ cup coconut oil.

Diarrhea

Sometimes caused by dietary indiscretion, diarrhea can also accompany a variety of illnesses. If your case is severe, or if it appears bloody or tarry looking, seek medical attention immediately. Keep hydrated, and let your doctor know if diarrhea is accompanied by a fever or if it lasts longer than 48 hours.

Helpful Essential Oils: frankincense, lemon, peppermint, Roman chamomile, tea tree, thyme

PEPPERMINT ABDOMINAL MASSAGE

TOPICAL, SAFE FOR CHILDREN AGES 6+

MUST HAVE Peppermint essential oil helps ease a long list of digestive complaints. It may help slow or stop diarrhea by easing intestinal muscle spasms, and it can help relieve uncomfortable abdominal cramping. MAKES ABOUT ¼ CUP

40 drops peppermint essential oil
¼ cup coconut oil, barely melted

1. In a glass jar with a tight-fitting lid, combine the peppermint essential oil and coconut oil. Using a thin utensil, such as a fork or butter knife, stir until well blended.

2. With your fingertips, apply a dime-size amount of the blend to your lower abdomen, using gentle, circular motions. Repeat every 2 to 3 hours until the diarrhea slows or stops.

3. Keep the blend in a cool, dark place between uses.

Tip: Create a synergistic blend by reducing the amount of peppermint essential oil to 20 drops and adding 10 drops each of Roman chamomile and thyme essential oils. In the jar, combine the essential oils and let them rest for about 1 hour before adding the coconut oil and completing the recipe.

SYNERGISTIC TUMMY RUB

TOPICAL, SAFE FOR CHILDREN AGES 2+

Soothing peppermint, lavender, and Roman chamomile essential oils deliver a relaxing fragrance that helps take your mind off discomfort, while the oils' antispasmodic and antibacterial properties get to work. MAKES ABOUT 2 TABLESPOONS

10 drops lavender essential oil
4 drops peppermint essential oil

8 drops Roman chamomile essential oil
2 tablespoons olive oil

1. In a small bottle or jar with a tight-fitting lid, combine the lavender, peppermint, and Roman chamomile essential oils. Let them rest for at least 1 hour.

2. Add the olive oil, cover the container, and shake well to combine.

3. With your fingertips, apply a dime-size amount of the blend to your lower abdomen, using gentle, circular motions. Repeat every 2 to 3 hours until the diarrhea slows or stops.

4. Keep the blend in a cool, dark place between uses.

   Tip: Make this blend safe for children under 2 years by reducing the peppermint essential oil to 1 drop or omitting it.

Earache

Using aromatherapy treatments at the first sign of an earache can sometimes prevent serious pain and fever from developing. *Do not put essential oils or other materials into your ear canals,* and see your doctor if your symptoms worsen.

Helpful Essential Oils: clove, eucalyptus, lavender, lemon, lemongrass, peppermint, rosemary, tea tree, thyme

TEA TREE–LEMONGRASS EAR POULTICE

TOPICAL, SAFE FOR CHILDREN AGES 2+

MUST HAVE Lemongrass and tea tree essential oils kill bacteria and relieve discomfort. This remedy calls for treating both ears, even if just one feels painful; treating both can help prevent earache from developing in the second ear. This is a useful strategy if your ear pain may be caused by moisture. MAKES ABOUT 6 TREATMENTS

4 drops lemongrass essential oil   1 tablespoon sweet almond oil
3 drops tea tree essential oil

1. In a small bottle with a tight-fitting lid, combine the lemongrass and tea tree essential oils. Let them rest for at least 1 hour before proceeding.

2. Add the sweet almond oil, cover the container, and shake well to combine.

3. Use 2 cotton balls and place about ¼ teaspoon of the blend on each. The cotton balls should be just barely moistened so no oil drips into the ear canals.

4. Place the cotton balls into the outer portions of the ears as you would earbuds. Relax and leave the cotton balls in place for at least 15 minutes. Repeat the treatment 2 to 3 times daily, continuing for at least 2 days after pain stops.

5. Keep the poultice in a cool, dark place between uses.

Tip: Sweet almond oil is ideal, as it is lightweight and absorbs quickly, but you can use any other carrier in a pinch.

LAVENDER HOT COMPRESS

TOPICAL, SAFE FOR CHILDREN AGES 6+

MUST HAVE Lavender essential oil can help stop an earache fast, particularly when you add heat to the equation. Be sure the water you use for this compress is comfortable to the touch, and wring out the cloth well so no moisture makes its way into the ear canal.

MAKES 1 TREATMENT

1 drop lavender essential oil	1 cup hot, but comfortable
4 drops carrier oil of choice	to the touch, water

1. In a small dish, combine the lavender essential oil and carrier oil.

2. Dip a cotton ball into the blend, squeeze out any excess to prevent dripping, and place it securely in the outer ear.

3. Fill a shallow bowl with the hot water and place a soft cloth in it to soak. Wring the excess water from the cloth. Fold it so it fits comfortably in your hand, and press it against the cotton ball

and ear area. When the cloth cools, repeat the moistening and wringing. Continue the treatment for at least 5 minutes and repeat 2 to 3 times daily.

4. Continue the treatments for at least 2 days after pain stops.

Tip: You can use a heating pad instead of a warm washcloth. Use the lowest setting and wrap it in a soft towel or clean T-shirt to keep it from coming into direct contact with your skin.

Eczema

Itching, redness, and inflammation make eczema a tough condition to live with, and it can be very difficult to keep yourself comfortable when symptoms flare. Always patch test essential oils carefully before using them to help with eczema; if you're sensitive, the oils could make matters worse instead of providing the comfort you need.

Helpful Essential Oils: frankincense, geranium, lavender, patchouli, peppermint, Roman chamomile, tea tree, thyme

PATCHOULI ROLL-ON

TOPICAL, SAFE FOR CHILDREN AGES 2+

Patchouli's healing and anti-inflammatory properties make it a favorite ingredient in aromatherapy treatments for eczema. If stress is a factor in your breakouts, you'll be glad to learn that patchouli helps your psyche, while improving your skin's condition. MAKES ABOUT 1 TABLESPOON

8 drops patchouli essential oil

1 tablespoon fractionated coconut oil

1. In a roller bottle, combine the patchouli essential oil and fractionated coconut oil. Cover the bottle and shake well to combine.

2. Dab a small amount on each affected area. Repeat as needed to combat itching and dryness throughout the day.

3. Keep the roll-on in a cool, dark place between applications.

Tip: Coconut oil has anti-inflammatory properties, and it works very well with patchouli and other eczema-fighting essential oils. Fractionated coconut oil remains liquid even at cool temperatures but you can make a similar remedy with regular coconut oil; you'll need to package the remedy in a small jar since it won't stay in liquid form.

SYNERGISTIC ECZEMA BALM

TOPICAL, SAFE FOR CHILDREN AGES 12+

Anti-inflammatory coconut oil combines with a synergistic blend of five essential oils, soothing compromised skin and helping it heal faster. MAKES ABOUT ¼ CUP

6 drops geranium essential oil

10 drops lavender essential oil

8 drops patchouli essential oil

12 drops Roman chamomile
essential oil

6 drops thyme essential oil

¼ cup organic coconut oil,
barely melted

1. In a small jar with a tight-fitting lid, combine the geranium, lavender, patchouli, Roman chamomile, and thyme essential oils. Let them rest for at least 1 hour before proceeding.

2. Using a thin utensil, such as a fork or butter knife, stir in the coconut oil until blended.

3. Apply a small dab of balm to each affected area, using just enough to cover. A drop or two should suffice. Repeat 2 to 3 times daily as needed.

4. Keep the balm in a cool, dark place between uses.

Tip: If preferred, create a liquid version of this remedy with fractionated coconut oil and package a small amount in a roller bottle for all-day portability.

Gingivitis

Swollen, inflamed gums that bleed each time you brush and floss are a sure sign you're suffering from gingivitis. It's vital to see your dentist for regular cleanings and other necessary treatments, but aromatherapy can provide comfort and help compromised gums heal between visits. Always continue your standard oral care; the importance of brushing, flossing, and rinsing can't be understated.

Helpful Essential Oils: clove, frankincense, grapefruit, lavender, lemon, lemongrass, peppermint, Roman chamomile, rosemary, thyme

PEPPERMINT-CLOVE OIL PULL

TOPICAL, SAFE FOR CHILDREN AGES 12+

MUST HAVE Peppermint and clove essential oils freshen breath naturally, while killing bacteria and promoting healing. If your gums are sore, these oils will provide some relief, and you might notice your teeth look whiter, too. MAKES ABOUT 24 TREATMENTS

2 drops clove essential oil   ½ cup coconut oil, barely melted
4 drops peppermint essential oil

1. In a jar with a tight-fitting lid, combine the clove and peppermint essential oils.

2. With a whisk or a thin utensil, such as a fork or butter knife, mix in the coconut oil to combine.

3. Each morning before eating or drinking anything, or each night before bed, place about 1 teaspoon of the oil-pulling blend in your mouth. Chew it until it melts, swish it around your mouth, and use suction to pull the oil blend between your teeth. Try to make each treatment last for at least 10 minutes.

4. When finished, spit the oil out into the trash (it'll clog drains). Rinse your mouth with fresh water and brush your teeth as usual.

5. Keep the blend in a cool, dark place between uses.

   Tip: If you're new to oil pulling, you may want to start with just a few minutes at a time. The practice feels strange at first, but you'll soon look forward to it.

LEMONGRASS MOUTH RINSE

TOPICAL, SAFE FOR CHILDREN 12+

MUST HAVE Lemongrass essential oil is powerful antimicrobial agent, and it has been studied for use in treating a variety of diseases. One study, published in the *Libyan Journal of Medicine,* showed that mouthwash containing lemongrass was effective in treating gingivitis. MAKES ABOUT 1 CUP

12 drops lemongrass essential oil   1 teaspoon baking soda
1 cup distilled water

1. In a bottle with a tight-fitting cap, combine the lemongrass essential oil, distilled water, and baking soda. Cover the bottle and shake well to dissolve the baking soda.

2. After brushing your teeth, rinse your mouth with approximately 1½ teaspoons of the rinse. Swish for at least 30 seconds before spitting it out into the sink. Repeat at least twice daily.

3. Keep the rinse in a cool, dark place between uses.

   Tip: If you don't have lemongrass essential oil, make this rinse with other gingivitis-fighting essential oils. Try a combination of peppermint, lemon, and clove for fresh breath and a pleasant tingle.

Hangover

A hangover is a sign your body is working hard to expel excess toxins. Aromatherapy helps make symptoms a bit easier to deal with, and, in some cases, may even eliminate discomfort altogether. Treat yourself to plenty of hydration and good nutrition, and try to get some rest if you can.

Helpful Essential Oils: clary sage, grapefruit, lavender, lemon, lemongrass, peppermint, Roman chamomile, rosemary, thyme

LEMON-PEPPERMINT SHOWER STEAM

AROMATIC, SAFE FOR CHILDREN 6+

MUST HAVE Peppermint and lemon essential oil help combat nausea and fatigue, while also providing headache relief. This refreshing shower steam will help you feel better quickly. Follow up with Rosemary-Grapefruit Temple Rub (page 114) for even better results. MAKES 1 TREATMENT

6 drops lemon essential oil   4 drops peppermint essential oil

1. Drip the essential oils onto the bottom of the shower, as far from the drain as possible. Cover the drain with a washcloth or hand towel.

2. Shower as usual, inhaling deeply. Add more drops to the if you'd like your treatment to last longer.

Tip: This remedy is also great for headaches and nausea not caused by hangovers, during cold season, or any time you need a pick-me-up.

ROSEMARY-GRAPEFRUIT TEMPLE RUB

AROMATIC, MAY CAUSE PHOTOSENSITIVITY, SAFE FOR CHILDREN 12+

Rosemary essential oil is a mild stimulant that clears your mind and reduces mental fatigue, while also helping with headache pain. Grapefruit aids with headaches, too, and it helps your body flush toxins faster. Applied to the temples, this simple treatment can make the "morning after" feel a bit brighter. MAKES ABOUT 1 TABLESPOON

8 drops grapefruit essential oil

12 drops rosemary essential oil

1 tablespoon fractionated coconut oil

1. In a roller bottle, combine the grapefruit and rosemary essential oils with the fractionated coconut oil. Cover the bottle and shake well to combine.

2. Dab a small amount on each temple. Repeat as needed to relieve hangover symptoms throughout the day.

3. Keep the roll-on in a cool, dark place between applications.

Tip: If you feel nauseated, add 4 to 6 drops peppermint essential oil to the blend.

Headache

A headache can make it tough to concentrate on important tasks, or even relax, leaving you in a frustrating limbo in which everything feels difficult. Aromatherapy can help, particularly when you start treatments as soon as you notice a headache coming on. If needed, use essential oils to complement over-the-counter pain medications.

Helpful Essential Oils: clove, eucalyptus, frankincense, grapefruit, lavender, lemon, lemongrass, peppermint, rosemary, thyme

SYNERGISTIC HEADACHE BALM

TOPICAL, SAFE FOR CHILDREN 12+

Lavender essential oil is a mild muscle relaxant that can work wonders on headaches caused by stress and tension, and it can sometimes stop migraines, too. Rosemary, peppermint, and thyme fight pain, while promoting increased circulation.

MAKES ABOUT 1 TABLESPOON

12 drops lavender essential oil

8 drops peppermint essential oil

8 drops rosemary essential oil

4 drops thyme essential oil

1 tablespoon fractionated coconut oil

1. In a roller bottle, combine the lavender, peppermint, rosemary, and thyme essential oils. Let them rest for about 1 hour.

2. Add the fractionated coconut oil, cap the bottle, and shake well to combine.

3. Dab a small amount on each temple and onto the base of your neck at the hairline. If you notice your headache is centered at a certain spot on your skull, apply a drop of balm there as well. Take a few minutes to relax and breathe deeply while the essential oils work. Repeat as needed.

4. Keep the roll-on in a cool, dark place between applications.

Tip: You can make a similar headache balm even if you're missing an oil or two, and experiment with different headache-fighting oils to see what works best for you.

PEPPERMINT-EUCALYPTUS TENSION TAMER

TOPICAL, SAFE FOR CHILDREN AGES 12+

MUST
HAVE Peppermint and eucalyptus essential oils increase circulation, ease inflammation, and relieve pain. Try this simple remedy next time you're suffering from a tension headache.

MAKES ABOUT 1 TABLESPOON

12 drops eucalyptus essential oil
10 drops peppermint essential oil

1 tablespoon fractionated coconut oil

1. In a roller bottle, combine the eucalyptus and peppermint essential oils. Let them rest for about 1 hour.

2. Add the fractionated coconut oil, cap the bottle, and shake well to combine.

3. Dab a small amount of the tension tamer across the hairline, both on the forehead and the base of your neck. If you notice your headache is centered at a certain spot on your skull, apply a drop of balm there as well. Take a few minutes to relax and breathe deeply while the essential oils work. Repeat as needed.

4. Keep the roll-on in a cool, dark place between applications.

Tip: This headache remedy is also a good choice for relieving sinus pain, simply apply a dab to each temple.

Heartburn

Heartburn occurs when stomach acid makes its way up into the esophagus and burns sensitive tissues. While aromatherapy can help you feel more comfortable, it's important to address underlying lifestyle issues that lead to heartburn. Some foods make it worse, and overeating, eating too close to bedtime, and excess alcohol can exacerbate the problem. If heartburn happens frequently, talk with your doctor.

Helpful Essential Oils: grapefruit, lavender, lemon, Roman chamomile

SYNERGISTIC HEARTBURN MASSAGE

TOPICAL, MAY CAUSE PHOTOSENSITIVITY, SAFE FOR AGES 12+

Grapefruit, lemon, lavender, and Roman chamomile essential oils provide a relaxing fragrance that can help take your mind off the painful, burning sensation, while the oils work to provide relief from discomfort. MAKES ABOUT 2 TABLESPOONS

14 drops grapefruit essential oil
8 drops lavender essential oil
8 drops lemon essential oil

8 drops Roman chamomile essential oil
2 tablespoons olive oil

1. In a small bottle or jar with a tight-fitting lid, combine the grapefruit, lavender, lemon, and Roman chamomile essential oils. Let them rest for at least 1 hour before continuing.

2. Add the olive oil, cover the container, and shake well to combine.

3. With your fingertips, apply a dime-size amount of the blend to your upper abdomen, using gentle, circular motions. Repeat hourly, if needed; one application is often enough.

4. Keep the blend in a cool, dark place between uses.

   Tip: Try resting on your left side with your head and upper chest slightly elevated on a pillow for about 15 minutes after your massage. This can help bring your digestive system back into balance.

ROMAN CHAMOMILE STEAM

AROMATIC, SAFE FOR CHILDREN AGES 6+

MUST HAVE Roman chamomile essential oil helps stop heartburn, while promoting relaxation. This simple treatment is ideal for anyone who suffers from heartburn or general gastric distress, and it provides soothing relief from the stress that often accompanies abdominal pain. You can use Roman chamomile in the bath or shower, add it to an essential oil inhaler, wear aromatherapy jewelry, or use a diffuser for a similar effect. MAKES 1 TREATMENT

8 drops Roman chamomile essential oil

2 cups steaming water (not boiling)

1. In a large, shallow bowl, combine the Roman chamomile essential oil and the hot water.

2. Place the bowl on a towel-topped table, and sit comfortably in front of the bowl.

3. Breathe slowly and deeply over the bowl until the water cools. Repeat as needed.

Tip: This strong steam treatment isn't suitable for children under 6 years, but you can treat them to a similar aromatherapy experience by placing 2 to 3 drops of Roman chamomile essential oil in a warm bath and allowing them to soak for at least 10 minutes.

Hemorrhoids

Hemorrhoids are caused by varicose veins in the rectal area; they itch and burn, and they can be terribly painful. Aromatherapy treatments can bring comfort, but in most cases you'll need to address underlying issues to make the problem go away for good. Surgical intervention is sometimes the only option in severe or prolapsed hemorrhoids; talk to your doctor for a comprehensive healing plan.

Helpful Essential Oils: frankincense, geranium, lavender, patchouli, peppermint, Roman chamomile, tea tree

COOLING PEPPERMINT-TEA TREE HEMORRHOID WIPES

TOPICAL, SAFE FOR AGES 12+

MUST HAVE Peppermint and tea tree essential oils combine with witch hazel to soothe the pain and itch of hemorrhoids, while simultaneously easing swelling. This remedy calls for avocado oil, which also soothes inflammation; if you don't have it on hand, olive oil is a respectable stand-in. MAKES 20 TO 40 TREATMENTS

4 drops peppermint essential oil
8 drops tea tree essential oil
½ cup alcohol-free witch hazel

1 tablespoon avocado oil
1 package unscented flushable wipes

1. In a jar with a tight-fitting lid, combine the tea tree and peppermint essential oils. Let them rest for at least 1 hour.

2. Add the witch hazel and avocado oil, cover the container, and shake to combine.

3. Open the package of wipes and pour the contents of the jar into it. Close the package and massage it for a few seconds to be sure that all wipes are saturated.

4. Carefully dab the affected area with a wipe or two after each bowel movement, and follow up with a treatment of Soothing Lavender-Geranium Balm if you like. Repeat after bathing or showering, and again at bedtime. Continue using these wipes as needed.

5. Keep the package in a cool, dark place between uses.

Tip: If your hemorrhoids are bleeding, use the tea tree and peppermint essential oils in a soothing sitz bath. Add them to warm, shallow bathwater and soak for at least 10 minutes.

SOOTHING LAVENDER-GERANIUM BALM

TOPICAL, SAFE FOR AGES 12+

MUST HAVE Lavender and geranium essential oils help soothe and heal compromised tissue, while easing the pain, itching, and swelling. Coconut oil provides relief from inflammation. While you can use this remedy on its own, it works best when applied after a hemorrhoid-specific cleansing treatment, such as Cooling Peppermint–Tea Tree Hemorrhoid Wipes (page 119). This simple remedy works on a variety of rashes; it's also a good choice for dealing with eczema and insect bites. MAKES ABOUT ¼ CUP

10 drops geranium essential oil
20 drops lavender essential oil

¼ cup coconut oil, barely melted

1. In a jar with a tight-fitting lid, combine the lavender and geranium essential oils. Let them rest for at least 1 hour.

2. Using a thin utensil, such as a fork or butter knife, stir in the coconut oil to blend completely.

3. After cleansing, use a cotton cosmetic pad to apply a pea-size amount of the balm to the affected area. Repeat as needed throughout the day and just before bedtime. Continue use as often as needed.

4. Keep the balm in a cool, dark place between uses.

Tip: If you prefer to use a liquid carrier for this remedy, avocado, olive, and sesame oil are all good choices.

Indigestion

Gassiness, bloating, and a feeling of heaviness and distension are just some of the discomforts associated with indigestion. Aromatherapy encourages the smooth muscles lining the digestive tract to relax, easing abdominal pain, flatulence, and related symptoms.

Helpful Essential Oils: clove, lavender, peppermint, Roman chamomile, rosemary, thyme

SYNERGISTIC ABDOMINAL MASSAGE

TOPICAL, SAFE FOR CHILDREN AGES 6+

Crisp peppermint, warming thyme, soothing lavender, and calming Roman chamomile essential oils deliver a comforting fragrance that can help take your mind off digestive discomfort, while the oils' antispasmodic and muscle-relaxing properties address symptoms. A special circular massage technique helps stimulate your digestive tract and move things along. MAKES ABOUT 2 TABLESPOONS

6 drops lavender essential oil
4 drops peppermint essential oil
6 drops Roman chamomile
   essential oil

4 drops thyme essential oil
2 tablespoons olive oil

1. In a small bottle or jar with a tight-fitting lid, combine the lavender, peppermint, Roman chamomile, and thyme essential oils. Let them rest for at least 1 hour.

2. Add the olive oil, cover the container, and shake well to combine.

3. With your fingertips, apply a dime-size amount of the blend to your abdomen, using a little more or less as needed to cover the entire area.

4. Recline comfortably and take some deep, slow breaths while massaging your abdomen using firm, clockwise strokes. Continue massaging until you start to feel better. Repeat every 2 to 3 hours, if needed.

5. Keep the blend in a cool, dark place between uses.

Tip: You can make this blend safe for children under 6 years by omitting the thyme essential oil. For children under age 2 years, reduce the peppermint to 1 drop or omit it.

CLARY SAGE–CLOVE AROMATHERAPY STEAM

AROMATIC, SAFE FOR CHILDREN AGES 6+

Clary sage and clove help tight, uncomfortable abdominal muscles relax, while steam speeds delivery into your system. You can use this blend in a bath or shower, or add it to an essential oil inhaler, aromatherapy jewelry, or a diffuser. MAKES 1 TREATMENT

8 drops clary sage essential oil

3 drops clove essential oil

2 cups steaming hot water (not boiling)

1. In a large, shallow bowl, combine the clary sage and clove essential oils with the hot water.

2. Place the bowl on a towel-topped table, and sit comfortably in front of the bowl.

AROMATHERAPY FOR BEGINNERS

3. Breathe slowly and deeply over the bowl until the water cools. Repeat as needed.

Tip: If don't have clove or clary sage, try this with any digestive essential oils. Whether used singly or combined, they are can provide some relief.

Insect Bites and Bee Stings

Unless the weather is chilly, outdoor adventures tend to bring contact with biting insects. Essential oils can put a stop to the itching and stinging, and often reduce swelling while helping irritated skin heal. Aromatherapy is not a substitute for antihistamines; if you're allergic to bees, always keep essential prescriptions handy and check with your doctor to be certain it's okay to use essential oils to make yourself more comfortable after a bee sting.

Helpful Essential Oils: clove, eucalyptus, lavender, patchouli, peppermint, Roman chamomile, tea tree, thyme

LAVENDER-TEA TREE NEAT TREATMENT

TOPICAL, SAFE FOR CHILDREN AGES 6+

MUST HAVE This simple, effective blend offers pain relief, while providing antiseptic, anti-inflammatory, and sedative effects. Lavender and tea tree essential oils help prevent infection, plus they offer immediate help with itching and stinging.

MAKES ABOUT 40 TREATMENTS

20 drops lavender essential oil   20 drops tea tree essential oil

1. In a small glass bottle with a dropper or orifice reducer, combine the lavender and tea tree essential oils. Let them rest for at least 1 hour before use.

2. Apply a drop of the blend to a cotton ball or swab, and gently dab each bite.

3. Repeat 2 to 3 times daily until bites are no longer sore or itchy.

4. Keep the bottle in a cool, dark place between uses.

   Tip: If you have sensitive skin or want to treat a child younger than 6 years with this blend, use just 15 drops of each essential oil and mix with ¼ cup of your favorite carrier oil.

PEPPERMINT-THYME SPRAY

TOPICAL, SAFE FOR CHILDREN AGES 6+

Peppermint and thyme essential oils offer strong medicinal action, helping to keep bug bites clean and preventing infection, while soothing the itch. Witch hazel and aloe add cooling power, and help prevent inflammation. MAKES ABOUT ½ CUP

20 drops peppermint essential oil	½ cup alcohol-free witch hazel
10 drops thyme essential oil	1 teaspoon aloe vera gel

1. In a bottle fitted with a spray top, combine the peppermint and thyme essential oils. Let them rest for at least 1 hour.

2. Add the witch hazel and aloe vera gel, cap the bottle, and shake well to combine. Shake again before each application.

3. Spritz each insect bite and allow the area to air-dry. Repeat every 2 to 3 hours as needed until the itching and pain subside.

4. Keep the spray in a cool, dark place between uses; refrigerate if you think you'd like even cooler relief.

   Tip: You can make this spray without witch hazel. White vinegar or apple cider vinegar provide relief from pain and itching, although the smell is not as pleasant. To make this remedy safe for children under 6 years, replace the thyme essential oil with lavender or clove.

AROMATHERAPY FOR BEGINNERS

Insomnia

Sleeplessness often plagues us when we need rest most. Luckily, aromatherapy can help you drift off to sleep, especially when you address lifestyle factors simultaneously. Treatments work best when you refrain from viewing TV, computer, and smartphone screens before lying down to sleep. Soothing music, dim lights, and herbal bedtime tea can intensify relaxation, so try those as well.

Helpful Essential Oils: clary sage, frankincense, lavender, patchouli, Roman chamomile

CLARY SAGE BEDTIME BALM

AROMATIC, SAFE FOR CHILDREN 12+

MUST HAVE Clary sage has a peaceful scent that might remind you of lavender once it has evaporated. It's an effective insomnia remedy by itself, but works well when combined with other relaxing essential oils. This remedy can be quite strong thanks to the natural muscle-relaxant properties of clary sage; it's best to use it right after you climb into bed. MAKES ABOUT 1 TABLESPOON

36 drops clary sage essential oil

1 tablespoon fractionated coconut oil

1. In a roller bottle, combine the clary sage oil and fractionated coconut oil. Cap the container and shake well to combine.

2. Dab a small amount on each temple. Dab another dot or two onto your chest. Relax and breathe deeply until you drift off to sleep.

3. Keep your balm in a cool, dark place between uses.

   Tip: If you'd like to use clary sage to help a child under 12 with insomnia, reduce the amount of essential oil to 8 drops and use the remedy as recommended. For children under age 6 years, try lavender essential oil instead.

AROMATIC, SAFE FOR ALL AGES

Clary sage, frankincense, lavender, patchouli, and Roman chamomile essential oils reduce stress and anxiety, while promoting a sense of peaceful calm. MAKES ABOUT 1 CUP

5 drops clary sage essential oil

2 drops frankincense essential oil

15 drops lavender essential oil

2 drops patchouli essential oil

10 drops Roman chamomile essential oil

1 cup water

1. In a bottle with a spray top, combine the clary sage, frankincense, lavender, patchouli, and Roman chamomile essential oils. Let them rest for at least 1 hour before proceeding.

2. Add the water, cap the bottle, and shake well before each use.

3. Mist your bedroom just before settling in. This spray isn't very strong; use as much as you like to create a pleasing atmosphere. Relax and breathe deeply while going through your bedtime routine.

4. Keep your bedtime spray in a cool, dark place between uses.

   Tip: You can create a similar spray even if you're missing an ingredient or two. You can also add a little more of whichever essential oils you prefer to create a customized scent.

Laryngitis

Laryngitis occurs when vocal cords are irritated and inflamed, sometimes causing a hoarse voice; other sufferers may lose their voices completely. Coughing, an itchy, dry feeling, and difficulty swallowing are other symptoms. While laryngitis usually clears up on its own, aromatherapy can bring comfort as you wait to recover. Check with your doctor if you are in pain or suspect an infection, and let your vocal cords rest while healing.

Helpful Essential Oils: clove, eucalyptus, frankincense, geranium, lavender, lemon, lemongrass, peppermint, Roman chamomile, rosemary, tea tree, thyme

CLOVE GARGLE

TOPICAL, SAFE FOR CHILDREN AGES 12+

MUST HAVE This gargle calls for simple ingredients, and provides fast, long-lasting relief. The sesame oil offers some anti-inflammatory benefits of its own, but if you don't have sesame oil on hand, use avocado oil or olive oil instead. MAKES ABOUT 1 CUP

8 drops clove essential oil   1 cup water
1 tablespoon sesame oil

1. In a jar or bottle with a tight-fitting lid, combine the clove essential oil, sesame oil, and water. Cover the container and shake well to combine thoroughly before each use.

2. Gargle with about 1½ teaspoons of the blend for 30 seconds to 1 minute. Repeat every 2 to 3 hours, as needed.

3. Keep your gargle in a cool, dark place between uses.

Tip: If you don't have clove essential oil on hand, you can obtain a bit of relief using 6 drops of lemon essential oil and 2 drops of peppermint essential oil in its place.

LEMONGRASS THROAT SPRAY

TOPICAL, SAFE FOR CHILDREN AGES 6+

MUST HAVE Lemongrass kills bacteria, helps prevent infection, offers strong pain relief and can help put a stop to itching and muscle spasms. MAKES ABOUT ½ CUP

20 drops lemongrass essential oil   7 tablespoons water
1 tablespoon vodka (optional)

1. In a bottle fitted with a spray top, combine the lemongrass essential oil, vodka (if using), and water. Cap the bottle and shake well before each use.

2. Tilt your head back slightly and open your mouth wide. Apply 2 to 3 spritzes to the back of your throat. Repeat as needed throughout each day while recovering.

3. Keep your throat spray in a cool, dark place between treatments; refrigerate it if you think you might like a colder sensation.

Tip: You can create a synergistic blend for laryngitis using any of the recommended essential oils. Add 6 drops of peppermint and 6 drops of clove essential oils to this spray if you'd like to try something different.

Menopause Symptoms

Aromatherapy won't stop the natural process of menopause, but it can help ease symptoms such as hot flashes, night sweats, and mood swings, making "the change" a bit easier to deal with. If you take prescription medication for your symptoms, check with your doctor to be sure that essential oils won't cause adverse side effects.

Helpful Essential Oils: clary sage, eucalyptus, geranium, grapefruit, lavender, lemon, patchouli, peppermint, Roman chamomile, thyme

CLARY SAGE NECK MASSAGE

TOPICAL, SAFE FOR AGES 12+

Clary sage essential oil provides impressive relief from menopause symptoms. You can use this treatment daily as a preventive measure, and you can apply it whenever you need.

MAKES ABOUT 1 TABLESPOON

18 drops clary sage essential oil

1 tablespoon fractionated coconut oil

1. In a roller bottle, combine the clary sage essential oil and fractionated coconut oil. Cap the bottle and shake well to combine.

2. Roll the bottle across the nape of your neck. Repeat as needed throughout the day, particularly in the late afternoon and evening when you're unwinding.

3. Keep the roll-on in a cool, dark place between applications.

Tip: If you're suffering from night sweats and insomnia, try this remedy at bedtime and while diffusing lavender and/or Roman chamomile essential oils. You may find your quality of sleep improves.

COOLING SYNERGISTIC SPRAY

TOPICAL, SAFE FOR AGES 12+

Hot flashes can be unbearable, but prescriptions may contain questionable ingredients, such as pregnant mares' urine, which can cause unwanted side effects. This natural spray contains peppermint to provide cool relief, plus clary sage and other oils that mimic estrogen's function; regular use can help combat a variety of unpleasant menopause symptoms. Evening primrose oil is an optional; it is useful in treating menopause symptoms.

MAKES ABOUT ¼ CUP

20 drops clary sage essential oil
18 drops geranium essential oil
18 drops lavender essential oil
20 drops peppermint essential oil
18 drops thyme essential oil

1 tablespoon evening primrose oil
(optional)
3 tablespoons alcohol-free
witch hazel

1. In a bottle fitted with a spray top, combine the clary sage, geranium, lavender, peppermint, and thyme essential oils. Let them rest for at least 1 hour.

2. Add the evening primrose oil (if using). Cap the bottle and shake or swirl to combine.

3. Add the witch hazel, recap the bottle, and shake well to combine; shake again before each use. Apply a spritz or two to the back of your neck whenever you feel a hot flash coming on. Repeat as often as needed.

4. Keep your spray in a cool, dark place between uses.

Tip: If you like, create a massage oil rather than a spray. Simply replace the witch hazel with your favorite carrier oil.

Menstrual Cramps

Most women have experienced painful menstrual cramps, and many rely on over-the-counter pain relievers. Aromatherapy offers natural relief from cramps as well as mood swings and anxiety. If you have to choose just one or two oils for menstrual cramps and/or PMS, consider clary sage or lavender—both are strong antispasmodics that also promote relaxation.

Helpful Essential Oils: clary sage, clove, eucalyptus, geranium, lavender, peppermint, Roman chamomile, rosemary, thyme

FOUR-OIL SYNERGY MASSAGE

TOPICAL, SAFE FOR AGES 12+

Clary sage, lavender, and thyme combine with Roman chamomile essential oil to ease cramps and promote blood flow, while also alleviating the emotional upset that often pops up during your cycle. MAKES ABOUT ½ CUP

20 drops clary sage essential oil
20 drops lavender essential oil
20 drops Roman chamomile
   essential oil

20 drops thyme essential oil
½ cup jojoba oil

1. In a bottle or jar with a tight-fitting lid, combine the clary sage, lavender, Roman chamomile, and thyme essential oils. Let them rest for at least 1 hour.

2. Add the jojoba oil, cover the container, and shake or swirl to blend thoroughly.

3. Massage approximately ¼ teaspoon of the blend into your lower abdomen once or twice daily during the week preceding your period, using a little more or less as needed to cover the area. Continue use while any cramping persists.

4. Keep the container in a cool, dark place between uses.

   Tip: You can make a similar massage oil even if you're missing ingredients; massaging with just one of these relaxing oils can make a difference for any discomfort.

SYNERGISTIC PAIN-RELIEF BATH

TOPICAL, SAFE FOR AGES 12+

Soothing clary sage, lavender, and Roman chamomile essential oils combine with fresh-scented geranium, easing pain and alleviating tension. The Epsom salt can help relieve your cramps, too. MAKES 1 TREATMENT

2 cups Epsom salt	4 drops lavender essential oil
2 drops clary sage essential oil	2 drops Roman chamomile
2 drops geranium essential oil	essential oil

1. Fill your bathtub with hot water, while adding the Epsom salt.

2. Add the clary sage, geranium, lavender, and Roman chamomile essential oils to the bathwater just before you get in.

3. Breathe deeply and relax for at least 15 minutes.

4. Follow up with an abdominal massage, if needed.

Tip: This is a very relaxing bath, consider enjoying it when you can nap afterward. It's ideal for use at bedtime, whether you're suffering from cramps or not.

Nail Fungus

Sometimes uncomfortable but often simply unsightly, nail fungus tends to affect toenails more often than fingernails. Be sure to address the root cause of nail fungus during and after treatment. Prolonged dampness, exposure to wet flooring, and wearing synthetic socks instead of natural fibers can encourage fungal growth.

Helpful Essential Oils: clove, lavender, lemon, lemongrass, patchouli, tea tree, rosemary, thyme

LEMONGRASS NAIL BALM

TOPICAL, SAFE FOR CHILDREN AGES 12+

MUST HAVE Lemongrass is a potent antifungal agent, and coconut oil also offers some antifungal action. MAKES ABOUT 1 TABLESPOON

18 drops lemongrass essential oil

1 tablespoon coconut oil, barely melted

1. In a small jar with a tight-fitting lid, combine the lemongrass essential oil and coconut oil.

2. Using a small, thin instrument, such as a chopstick, stir the oils together.

3. With a cotton swab, apply 1 or 2 drops to each affected toenail after washing and drying your feet. Allow the blend to absorb fully before putting on socks. Repeat twice daily until the fungus is gone.

4. Keep the balm in a cool, dark place between uses.

Tip: You can make this remedy safe for children between the ages of 6 and 12 years by using 8 drops of lemongrass essential oil instead of 18.

TEA TREE NEAT TREATMENT FOR NAIL FUNGUS

TOPICAL, SAFE FOR CHILDREN AGES 12+

MUST HAVE Tea tree essential oil is one of the best antifungal essential oils available, plus it offers antiseptic and pain-relieving properties. This treatment is a strong one; ideal for tackling tough cases. MAKES 1 TREATMENT

1 drop tea tree essential oil

1. Wash and dry your feet.

2. With a cotton swab, apply 1 drop of tea tree essential oil to the affected toenail. Let the essential oil absorb fully before putting on socks.

3. Repeat twice daily until the fungus is gone.

Tip: Use tea tree essential oil to prevent nail fungus as well. Blend 12 drops tea tree essential oil with 2 tablespoons of your favorite carrier and apply it once daily to clean, dry nails.

PMS

PMS is completely natural, but that doesn't make it any easier to deal with. Aromatherapy helps tame your inner dragon by alleviating moodiness and helping with symptoms such as hot flashes, cramping, and nausea.

Helpful Essential Oils: clary sage, frankincense, geranium, lavender, patchouli, Roman chamomile, rosemary, thyme

SYNERGISTIC PMS DIFFUSER BLEND

AROMATIC, SAFE FOR AGES 12+

Clary sage, geranium, lavender, patchouli, and Roman chamomile essential oils create a lovely scent that relaxes your body and mind. Make this blend ahead of time and allow it to mature for at least a few days, if possible. MAKES ABOUT 30 TREATMENTS

20 drops clary sage essential oil

8 drops geranium essential oil

20 drops lavender essential oil

4 drops patchouli essential oil

20 drops Roman chamomile essential oil

1. In a dark-colored glass bottle with a dropper or orifice reducer, combine the clary sage, geranium, lavender, patchouli, and Roman chamomile essential oils. Let them rest for at least 1 hour.

2. Add 3 or 4 drops of the PMS blend to a diffuser and use according to the manufacturer's instructions. Repeat as needed.

3. Keep your diffuser blend in a cool, dark place between uses.

Tip: This diffuser blend is very relaxing. If you need to focus, add 8 to 10 drops of rosemary essential oil to the blend, or simply add a drop or two of rosemary to your diffuser along with the blended essential oils.

TENSION-TAMING ROLL-ON BLEND

TOPICAL, SAFE FOR AGES 12+

MUST HAVE Lavender, patchouli, and rosemary essential oils mingle to create an enticing, earthy fragrance that calms tension, while keeping you focused. This blend is ideal for combating PMS symptoms, and it's just the thing to relieve stress or anxiety. MAKES ABOUT 1 TABLESPOON

12 drops lavender essential oil

2 drops patchouli essential oil

4 drops rosemary essential oil

1 tablespoon fractionated coconut oil

1. In a roller bottle, combine the lavender, patchouli, and rosemary essential oils. Let them rest for about 1 hour.

2. Add the fractionated coconut oil, cap the bottle, and shake well to combine.

3. Dab a small amount on each temple. Take a few minutes to relax and breathe deeply. Repeat as needed.

4. Keep the roll-on in a cool, dark place between applications.

Tip: You can make a similar roll-on with any essential oils indicated for PMS. Experimentation is fun, and it will help you learn which oils are most effective for you.

Rashes

Poison ivy and its relatives cause nasty rashes, and so do certain chemicals. Even stress can bring on a case of hives. Fortunately, essential oils can help with pain and redness, often shortening a rash's duration. Always conduct a patch test with any essential oil you plan to use on a rash; if you're sensitive, aromatherapy may make matters worse.

Helpful Essential Oils: eucalyptus, frankincense, geranium, lavender, patchouli, peppermint, Roman chamomile, tea tree

TEA TREE-GERANIUM BALM

TOPICAL, SAFE FOR CHILDREN AGES 2+

MUST HAVE Tea tree and geranium essential oils soothe troubled skin, and coconut oil provides relief from inflammation. This simple remedy works on a variety of rashes; it's also great for dealing with eczema and insect bites. MAKES ABOUT ½ CUP

10 drops geranium essential oil
10 drops tea tree essential oil

½ cup organic coconut oil, barely melted

1. In a jar with a tight-fitting lid, combine the geranium and tea tree essential oils. Let them rest for at least 1 hour before proceeding.

2. Using a thin utensil, such as a fork or butter knife, stir in the coconut oil until well blended.

3. With your fingertips or a cotton pad, apply a pea-size amount of balm to each affected area, using a little more or less as needed to create a thin layer. Repeat as needed throughout the day, and continue use until the rash subsides.

4. Keep the balm in a cool, dark place between uses.

   Tip: You can create a similar balm with any rash-fighting essential oil. Try combining lavender with eucalyptus or tea tree, or consider a blend of lavender and peppermint. Soothing Lavender-Geranium Balm (page 120) is also a healing treatment that is great for rashes.

ANTI-ITCH BATH

TOPICAL, SAFE FOR CHILDREN AGES 2+

MUST HAVE Colloidal oatmeal is an excellent remedy for itchy rashes, so it's often sold in convenient premeasured packets. Lavender, peppermint, and tea tree essential oils help soothe the itch and take your mind off your troubles. MAKES 1 TREATMENT

1 packet colloidal oatmeal bath	2 drops peppermint essential oil
2 drops lavender essential oil	2 drops tea tree essential oil

1. Fill the bathtub with warm water and add the colloidal oatmeal.

2. Add the lavender, peppermint, and tea tree essential oils just before stepping into the tub. Relax for at least 15 minutes.

3. Pat yourself dry and follow up with Soothing Lavender-Geranium Balm (page 120), if you like.

Tip: If you want to save money on colloidal oatmeal, you can make your own by adding 4 cups rolled oats to a food processer or high-powered blender, and grind it into a fine powder. Use ½ cup of colloidal oatmeal per bath.

Ringworm and Jock Itch

Ringworm and jock itch are caused by tinea, which is actually a type of fungus, not a worm. The rash has a circular shape, raised edges, and blister-like lesions that sometimes break open and form a crust. This fungal infection is highly contagious, so personal hygiene is a vital part of treatment. Check with your doctor if your symptoms persist or worsen; some cases call for pharmaceutical treatment.

Helpful Essential Oils: clove, lavender, lemon, lemongrass, patchouli, tea tree, rosemary, thyme

QUICK CLOVE LOTION

TOPICAL, SAFE FOR CHILDREN AGES 12+

MUST HAVE Clove essential oil is an outstanding antifungal agent, and this simple remedy is quick and easy to make. If you have multiple patches of ringworm or jock itch, use an individual cotton swab to treat each one. MAKES ABOUT 2 TABLESPOONS

36 drops clove essential oil

2 tablespoons fragrance-free lotion

1. In a small bowl, combine the clove essential oil and lotion. Use a small whisk or a fork to blend. Transfer the lotion to a bottle or jar with a tight-fitting lid.

2. With cotton swabs, apply 1 or 2 drops of lotion to each affected area. Do not touch the swabs to unaffected skin, and dispose of them immediately after use.

3. Allow each treated area to dry before dressing. Repeat the treatment 2 to 3 times daily, continuing for 2 to 3 days after the lesions disappear.

4. Keep the lotion in a cool, dark place between uses.

Tip: You can use a similar treatment for children under age 12 years; reduce the amount of clove essential oil to 16 drops for children between the ages of 6 and 12, and to 8 drops for those between the ages of 2 and 6 years.

SYNERGISTIC ANTIFUNGAL BALM

TOPICAL, SAFE FOR CHILDREN AGES 6+

This soothing balm contains clove, lemongrass, tea tree, and thyme essential oil—four of the strongest antifungal oils available. Coconut oil also offers antifungal properties, plus it soothes itching and facilitates healing. MAKES ABOUT 2 TABLESPOONS

5 drops lemongrass essential oil	5 drops thyme essential oil
5 drops clove essential oil	2 tablespoons organic coconut
5 drops tea tree essential oil	oil, barely melted

1. In a jar with a tight-fitting lid, combine the clove, lemongrass, tea tree, and thyme essential oils. Let the blend rest for at least 1 hour.

2. Using a thin utensil, such as a chopstick, stir in the coconut oil to combine.

3. With cotton swabs, apply 1 or 2 drops of balm to each affected area. Do not touch the swabs to unaffected skin, and dispose of them immediately after use.

4. Allow each treated area to dry before dressing. Repeat the treatment 2 to 3 times daily, continuing for 2 to 3 days after the lesions disappear.

5. Keep the balm in a cool, dark place between uses.

Tip: You can make this balm even if you're missing some of the essential oils. Aim for a total of 20 drops of essential oil, and use up to 72 drops total if the person being treated is an adult.

Sinusitis

The sinus irritation that accompanies allergies, colds and flu, and upper respiratory infections can cause serious pain and lead to nagging headaches. Aromatherapy soothes tissues and kills pathogens. Serious cases of sinusitis often call for treatment with antibiotics, check in with your doctor if such is the case. If you opt for conventional treatment, it's likely you can continue to use aromatherapy to soothe your symptoms, while the antibiotics work on your infection from the inside out.

Helpful Essential Oils: clary sage, clove, eucalyptus, frankincense, geranium, lavender, lemon, lemongrass, peppermint, Roman chamomile, rosemary, tea tree, thyme

ROSEMARY-LEMON SINUS STEAM

AROMATIC, SAFE FOR CHILDREN AGES 6+

MUST HAVE Rosemary and lemon essential oils reduce sinus inflammation and kill bacteria, making it easier for your body to fight infection, while helping you feel more comfortable. If you like, use the blend in an essential oil inhaler, aromatherapy jewelry, or a diffuser. MAKES 1 TREATMENT

4 drops lemon essential oil

4 drops rosemary essential oil

2 cups steaming hot water (not boiling)

1. In a large, shallow bowl, combine lemon and rosemary essential oils with the hot water.

2. Place the bowl on a towel-topped table, and sit comfortably in front of the bowl.

3. Breathe slowly and deeply over the bowl until the water cools. Repeat as needed.

   Tip: This strong steam treatment isn't suitable for children under 6 years, but you can treat them to a similar aromatherapy experience by placing the essential oils in a warm bath and allowing them to soak for at least 10 minutes.

LAVENDER-TEA TREE NETI POT TREATMENT

TOPICAL, SAFE FOR CHILDREN AGES 12+

MUST HAVE Flushing your sinuses with a neti pot might seem challenging, but it provides tremendous relief from blocked and painful sinuses. This treatment calls for essential oils and a saline solution, plus a neti pot, which is usually easy to find at pharmacies or online. MAKES 1 TREATMENT

1 teaspoon natural Himalayan salt, or unprocessed sea salt

2 cups warm distilled water (body temperature or just a little bit warmer)

1 drop lavender essential oil

1 drop tea tree essential oil

1. In a clean liquid measuring cup, dissolve the salt in the warm water.

2. Add the lavender and tea tree essential oils.

3. Fill the neti pot as according to the instructions that accompany it.

4. Position yourself near a sink and bend over it with your head tilted to one side.

5. Hold your breath and pour the solution from the neti pot through the upper nostril. Allow the solution to flow through the lower nostril into the sink.

6. After the solution drains, refill the neti pot and repeat steps 4 and 5 with the other nostril.

7. Repeat at least 3 times daily while recovering from sinusitis. Make a fresh batch of saline each time you do the treatment.

   Tip: Not sure how to use a neti pot? You can find tutorials on YouTube.

Sprains and Strains

Mild sprains and strains can benefit from aromatherapy treatments alongside traditional remedies such as rest, ice, compression, and elevation. Fractures and serious sprains require emergency medical treatment; if you have even the slightest doubt, see your doctor immediately instead of reaching for the essential oils.

Helpful Essential Oils: clary sage, clove, eucalyptus, grapefruit, lavender, lemon, lemongrass, peppermint, Roman chamomile

SYNERGISTIC SPRAIN GEL

TOPICAL, SAFE FOR CHILDREN AGES 12+

Peppermint, Roman chamomile, and rosemary essential oils speed healing, while helping ease some of the pain that accompanies a sprain. If you have sprained a large joint, you may want to double or triple this recipe so you only have to blend it once. If you use arnica gel, you'll get even more pain relief. MAKES ABOUT 2 TABLESPOONS

16 drops peppermint essential oil

16 drops Roman chamomile essential oil

16 drops rosemary essential oil

2 tablespoons arnica gel, or aloe vera gel

1. In a small jar with a tight-fitting lid, combine the peppermint, Roman chamomile, and rosemary essential oils. Let the blend rest for at least 1 hour.

2. Using a thin utensil, such as a chopstick, stir in your gel of choice until all ingredients are completely combined.

3. With your fingers, apply a dime-size amount to the sprained area, using a little more or less as needed to cover the entire area.

4. Apply dressings or bandages, if needed, and rest with your sprained body part elevated, if possible.

5. Keep your gel in a cool, dry, place, or refrigerate it if you'd like a cooler sensation.

   Tip: You can formulate a similar gel with any of the indicated essential oils. All provide some relief; experimentation can help you determine which one(s) works best for your individual pain-management needs.

ROMAN CHAMOMILE-CLOVE MASSAGE OIL

TOPICAL, SAFE FOR CHILDREN AGES 12+

Roman chamomile and clove essential oils ease pain and promote faster healing. This balm is ideal for use while an older injury is healing. It encourages circulation and helps reduce inflammation, supporting your body's natural repair processes.

MAKES ABOUT ¼ CUP

20 drops clove essential oil

20 drops Roman chamomile essential oil

¼ cup jojoba oil

1. In a small bottle with a tight-fitting lid, combine the clove and Roman chamomile essential oils. Let them rest for at least 1 hour.

2. Add the jojoba oil, cap the bottle, and shake or swirl to combine the ingredients.

3. With your fingers, apply a dime-size amount of massage oil to the affected area, using a little more or less as needed. Massage gently, using circular motions. This may be a little uncomfortable, but it should not hurt. If you're still in pain, just lightly stroke the massage oil onto the injured area and allow it to penetrate without massaging. Repeat once or twice daily while healing.

4. Keep your massage oil in a cool, dark place between uses.

Tip: Jojoba oil is a good choice as it is light and penetrates quickly. Use another carrier, though, if you prefer.

Sunburn

We need a little bit of sun exposure to manufacture vitamin D, but overdoing it—even a little—can lead to sunburn. Aromatherapy treatments can bring comfort fast, and if you apply them as soon as you notice you've been burned, they can sometimes prevent blistering and peeling. If you have a deep, serious sunburn, see your doctor for emergency treatment.

Helpful Essential Oils: eucalyptus, frankincense, geranium, lavender, patchouli, peppermint, Roman chamomile, tea tree

LAVENDER SUNBURN GEL

TOPICAL, SAFE FOR CHILDREN AGES 2+

MUST HAVE   Aloe vera hydrates sunburned skin, while lavender essential oil promotes rapid healing. Look for pure aloe gel, with no alcohol, dyes, or other additives. MAKES ABOUT ½ CUP

20 drops lavender essential oil   ½ cup aloe vera gel

1. In a small bowl, combine the lavender essential oil and the aloe vera gel. With a small whisk or fork, stir until well combined. Transfer the blend to a container with a tight-fitting lid. A plastic squeeze-type travel bottle is ideal for this remedy.

2. Apply a generous amount of gel to each burned area. The exact amount will vary depending on the size of the area being treated.

3. Allow the treated skin to air-dry before dressing. Repeat as needed, at least 2 to 3 times daily while recovering.

4. Keep the sunburn gel in a cool, dark place between treatments, or refrigerate it for a cooling effect.

Tip: You can easily make this remedy in an existing container of aloe vera gel. Note the number of fluid ounces of gel inside the container and calculate the amount of lavender to use: Based on our formula here of 20 drops to ½ cup (4 fluid ounces), a 12-fluid ounce container would call for three times the amount of lavender, or 60 drops. After adding the lavender, cover the container and shake well to ensure it is combined.

SYNERGISTIC SUNBURN SPRAY

TOPICAL, SAFE FOR CHILDREN AGES 6+

This spray contains aloe for moisture along with Roman chamomile, frankincense, and lavender essential oils to soothe and heal skin, plus peppermint and tea tree to reduce pain. Witch hazel contributes its own anti-inflammatory effects, and imparts a cool, comforting tingle. MAKES ABOUT ½ CUP

10 drops frankincense essential oil
10 drops lavender essential oil
6 drops peppermint essential oil
10 drops Roman chamomile

4 drops tea tree essential oil
7 tablespoons alcohol-free witch hazel
1 tablespoon aloe vera gel

1. In a bottle fitted with a spray tip, combine the frankincense, lavender, peppermint, Roman chamomile, and tea tree essential oils. Let them rest for at least 1 hour.

2. Add the witch hazel and aloe vera gel, cap the bottle, and shake well to combine before each use.

3. Apply a light mist of spray to each burned area. Allow the area to dry before dressing. Repeat as often as needed.

4. Keep the spray in a cool, dry place between uses, or refrigerate it for a cooling effect.

Tip: This blend makes a nice skin toner for use after sun exposure, even if you haven't burned yourself.

Toothache

Although dental pain should always be addressed by a dentist, there are some times when it's necessary to wait for an appointment. Aromatherapy treatments help dull the ache in your mouth, while killing bacteria that can make infections worse.

Helpful Essential Oils: clove, lemongrass, peppermint, Roman chamomile, tea tree

CLOVE NEAT TREATMENT

TOPICAL, SAFE FOR CHILDREN AGES 12+

MUST HAVE Clove contains a natural numbing agent, while offering outstanding antibacterial action. This remedy works fast and provides long-lasting pain relief. MAKES 1 TREATMENT

1 drop clove essential oil

1. Place 1 drop of clove essential oil onto a cotton ball or cotton swab.

2. Open your mouth wide while looking in a mirror. Carefully position the swab or cotton ball alongside the sore tooth. Bite down gently to keep the cotton in place. Leave it in position for about 1 minute. Remove and discard the cotton ball. Repeat every 12 hours, or as needed.

Tip: If you don't have clove essential oil, try this with Roman chamomile instead. Blend 1 drop Roman chamomile essential oil with 1 drop carrier oil, such as coconut oil, which is a great choice for dental health, and follow the same instructions for application.

PAIN-RELIEVING OIL PULL

TOPICAL, SAFE FOR CHILDREN AGES 12+

Clove, lemongrass, and Roman chamomile essential oils combine with coconut oil, to kill bacteria while stopping pain. This is a milder treatment than the Clove Neat Treatment (page 145), but it still offers a good level of pain control. MAKES ABOUT 24 TREATMENTS

8 drops clove essential oil

4 drops lemongrass essential oil

4 drops Roman chamomile essential oil

½ cup coconut oil, barely melted

1. In a jar with a tight-fitting lid, combine the clove, lemongrass, and Roman chamomile essential oils. Let them rest for at least 1 hour.

2. With a whisk or a thin utensil, such as a fork or butter knife, stir in the coconut oil until well combined.

3. Place about 1 teaspoon of the oil-pulling blend in your mouth. Chew it until it melts, and swish it around your mouth, using suction to pull the oil blend between your teeth, for at least 10 minutes.

4. When finished, spit the oil into the trash (it'll clog drains). Rinse your mouth with fresh water and brush your teeth as usual. Repeat as needed to control oral pain while waiting for your dental appointment.

   Tip: If you're new to oil pulling, you may want to start with just a few minutes at a time.

Yeast Infection

Caused by the fungus *Candida*, yeast infections are itchy and uncomfortable. Antifungal essential oils can help, and are most effective when you begin treating the problem as soon as symptoms appear. Check with your doctor if your symptoms don't respond to aromatherapy. *Never use aromatherapy for yeast infections during pregnancy.*

Helpful Essential Oils: clove, frankincense, geranium, lavender, lemongrass, patchouli, rosemary, tea tree, thyme

LEMONGRASS-CLOVE COMPRESS

TOPICAL

MUST HAVE Lemongrass and clove essential oils offer strong antifungal action, while soothing the itch. Be certain you have conducted patch tests before applying this remedy to sensitive vaginal tissues.

MAKES ABOUT 2 TABLESPOONS

6 drops clove essential oil
18 drops lemongrass essential oil

2 tablespoons fractionated coconut oil

1. In a small jar with a tight-fitting lid, combine the clove and lemongrass essential oils with the fractionated coconut oil. Cover the container and shake or swirl to blend thoroughly.

2. Coat an applicator-free tampon in the mixture and insert it into the vagina per the manufacturer's instructions. Leave the compress in place for about 30 minutes. Remove and discard it. Repeat every 8 to 12 hours while symptoms persist, and for 2 to 3 days after the infection subsides.

3. Keep your oil blend in a cool, dark place between uses.

Tip: You can use any blend of the indicated essential oils to create a similar compress. A little goes a long way here; dilution rates between 3 and 4 percent should be adequate.

SOOTHING COCONUT SUPPOSITORIES

TOPICAL

These suppositories make short work of yeast infections, thanks to antifungal lavender, lemongrass, Roman chamomile, and tea tree essential oils. Coconut oil offers antifungal action, too, and its ability to melt at body temperature makes it the ideal carrier. Be certain you have conducted patch tests before applying this remedy to sensitive vaginal tissues. MAKES ABOUT 12 TREATMENTS

6 drops lavender essential oil
6 drops lemongrass essential oil
6 drops Roman chamomile
essential oil

6 drops tea tree essential oil
¼ cup organic coconut oil, melted

1. In a liquid measuring cup, combine the lavender, lemongrass, Roman chamomile, and tea tree essential oils with the melted coconut oil. Quickly transfer the liquid to a clean, dry ice-cube tray, placing about ½ inch of the blend into each of 12 compartments.

2. Place the tray into the freezer and check on it after about 10 minutes. It shouldn't take long for the coconut oil to solidify.

3. Insert a suppository into your vagina every 8 to 12 hours while the yeast infection persists, and continue for 2 to 3 days after symptoms subside.

4. Keep the remedy in the freezer so the suppositories don't melt.

   Tip: Melting oil can be messy. It's a good idea to protect your undergarments with panty liners while using this treatment.

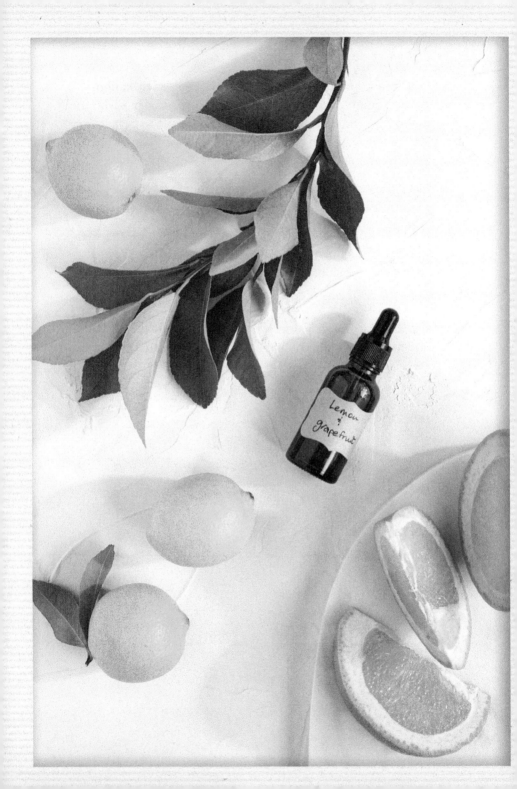

CHAPTER 6

Recipes for Personal Care and Emotional Well-Being

A romatherapy products are sold at a variety of stores, often a higher price than products with artificial fragrances. The recipes in this chapter are an introduction to making your own, far less expensive body care products. You'll discover just how easy it is to create beautifully scented bath and body solutions such as shampoos, conditioners, and lotions.

Emotional well-being and aromatherapy go hand in hand. Whether you need to calm turbulent anger, recover from emotional upset, or reduce stress, you'll find 20 suggested healing solutions here. Once you are familiar with essential oils and know which blends you like best, you can easily add emotional-healing properties to any of your personal care products to enjoy multiple benefits.

Acne

Almost everybody suffers from acne at some point. While severe cases may call for medical intervention, most clogged pores, blackheads, whiteheads, and pimples respond well to essential oils. Conduct patch tests before using new essential oils, especially on irritated, compromised skin, and consider whether you'll be spending time in the sun when deciding whether to use oils that can cause photosensitivity: The last thing you want is a sunburn.

Helpful Essential Oils: clove, eucalyptus, frankincense, grapefruit, lavender, lemon, lemongrass, patchouli, Roman chamomile tea tree, thyme

LEMONGRASS-TEA TREE TONER

TOPICAL, SAFE FOR CHILDREN AGES 12+

MUST HAVE Lemongrass and tea tree essential oils make short work of bacteria, while helping skin heal faster. The witch hazel in this toner offers a pleasant, cooling sensation. MAKES ½ CUP

8 drops lemongrass essential oil   ½ cup alcohol-free witch hazel
6 drops tea tree essential oil

1. In a bottle or jar with a tight-fitting lid, combine the lemongrass and tea tree essential oils. Let them rest for at least 1 hour.

2. Add the witch hazel, cover the container, and stir or shake well to combine completely. Shake again before each use.

3. With a cotton ball or cosmetic pad, apply about ¼ teaspoon of the toner to your freshly washed face, or other areas where acne is a problem. Use a little more or less as needed. Repeat 2 to 3 times daily while acne is visible, and continue using once daily as a preventive measure. Follow up with an oil-free moisturizer.

4. Keep the toner in a cool, dark place between uses.

Tip: This toner is easy to customize with any acne-fighting essential oils you have on hand. You can make it with a single oil or create new combinations.

TEA TREE NEAT TREATMENT FOR ACNE

TOPICAL, SAFE FOR CHILDREN AGES 12+

MUST HAVE When you feel a pimple forming and want to prevent it from getting worse, a dab of tea tree essential oil can help. And its ability to kill bacteria is ideal for existing blemishes.

MAKES 1 TREATMENT

1 drop tea tree essential oil

1. Wash and dry the affected area.

2. Use a cotton swab to apply a dab of tea tree essential oil to the blemish. Repeat once or twice daily until healed.

Tip: If you don't have tea tree essential or, or if it bothers you, use neat lavender or eucalyptus essential oil for a similar effect.

Aging Skin Care

Aging skin requires special care; fine lines and wrinkles, age spots, and dryness are normal signs that our skin's needs are changing. Aromatherapy supports healthy skin in many ways: Some oils encourage collagen production, others deliver antioxidants, and yet others help retain moisture.

Helpful Essential Oils: clary sage, frankincense, geranium, patchouli, Roman chamomile, thyme

MOISTURIZING OIL CLEANSE

TOPICAL, SAFE FOR AGES 12+

MUST HAVE Frankincense's nourishes skin to reduce signs of aging, making it an ally in your quest to keep skin looking vibrant. Oil cleansing removes impurities, while providing your skin with penetrating moisture. MAKES ABOUT ½ CUP

24 drops frankincense essential oil	½ cup avocado oil

1. In a bottle or jar with a tight-fitting lid, combine the frankincense essential oil and avocado oil.

2. Wet your face with warm water.

3. With your fingertips, apply about ½ teaspoon of the oil blend to your face. Massage using light, circular motions.

4. Soak a washcloth in warm water and wring out the excess. Place the cloth over your face for about 15 seconds. Use it to gently remove any excess oil.

5. With a soft towel, pat your skin dry. Repeat once or twice daily.

6. Keep the blend in a cool, dark place between uses.

Tip: You can use this blend to treat any area where dryness, sagging, or scaly skin is a problem.

ULTRA-MOISTURIZING FACIAL CREAM

TOPICAL, SAFE FOR AGES 12+

Roman chamomile essential oil reduces flakiness and inflammation, healing damage while restoring suppleness. This blend includes clary sage, frankincense, and geranium to help reduce visual signs of aging. The addition of apricot kernel oil and coconut oil, two carriers that provide deep moisture, helps to rejuvenate skin and fight free radicals. MAKES ABOUT 1 CUP

10 drops clary sage essential oil

10 drops frankincense
essential oil

5 drops geranium essential oil

10 drops Roman chamomile
essential oil

½ cup unrefined shea butter

½ cup coconut oil

1½ teaspoons apricot kernel oil

1½ teaspoons rosehip oil
(optional)

1 tablespoon vegetable glycerin
(optional)

1. In an 8-ounce or larger dark-colored glass bottle with a tight-fitting lid, combine the clary sage, frankincense, geranium, and Roman chamomile essential oils. Let them rest overnight.

2. In the clean, dry bowl of a blender or food processor, combine the essential oil blend, shea butter, coconut oil, apricot kernel oil, and rosehip oil and glycerin (if using). Process until smooth. Transfer the blend to a clean, dry mixer bowl, and refrigerate until firm.

3. With the whip or whisk attachment of a stand mixer or hand-held electric mixer, process the blend until it has a light, silky texture. Transfer the finished cream to a jar with a tight-fitting lid.

4. After washing your face, use your fingers to apply a pea-size amount of moisturizer. Use a little more or less as needed. Repeat once or twice daily.

5. Store the cream in a cool, dark place between uses; if it gets warm, it'll turn back into liquid. You can still use the cream this way, but the texture isn't as nice.

Tip: What is vegetable glycerin? Colorless, odorless, and highly moisturizing, glycerin is a blend of triglycerides sourced from oily plants such as soy and coconut. It acts as an emulsifier, helping to bind all the ingredients and delivering a pleasant texture.

Anxiety

Many of us experience occasional anxiety. Aromatherapy can help quiet your mind when anxious thoughts take over, and produce physical calming responses to slow your breathing and heart rate. Some can even help bring your blood pressure down a bit.

Helpful Essential Oils: clary sage, clove, frankincense, geranium, lemon, lavender, patchouli, rosemary, thyme

ANTI-ANXIETY DIFFUSER BLEND

AROMATIC, SAFE FOR ALL AGES

Clary sage, lavender, lemon, and patchouli essential oils deliver a delightful scent, while promoting calm. This intoxicating blend can be used in aromatherapy jewelry or essential oil inhalers, as well as added to bath products. MAKES ABOUT 30 TREATMENTS

30 drops clary sage essential oil

30 drops lavender essential oil

30 drops lemon essential oil

10 drops patchouli essential oil

1. In a dark-colored glass bottle with a dropper or orifice reducer, combine the clary sage, lavender, lemon, and patchouli essential oils. Let them rest for at least 1 hour.

2. Add 3 or 4 drops of the blend to a diffuser and use according to the manufacturer's instructions. Repeat any time anxious thoughts intrude.

3. Keep your diffuser blend in a cool, dark place between uses.

Tip: You can use this blend while resting, meditating, or doing another activity that takes your mind off your troubles. You'll soon associate the scent with relaxing activities and enjoy faster relief from anxiety.

ANTI-ANXIETY ROLL-ON

TOPICAL, SAFE FOR CHILDREN AGES 12+

Frankincense, lavender, and Roman chamomile essential oil create a pleasant, balanced scent, while alleviating feelings of anxiety. This blend is great for softening skin, too. MAKES ABOUT 1 TABLESPOON

4 drops frankincense essential oil

4 drops lavender essential oil

4 drops Roman chamomile essential oil

1 tablespoon fractionated coconut oil

1. In a roller bottle, combine the lavender, Roman chamomile, and frankincense essential oils. Let them rest for at least 1 hour.

2. Add the fractionated coconut oil, cap the bottle, and shake well to combine.

3. Dab a small amount on each temple. If you like, also apply the blend to your inner wrists or other pulse points. Repeat as needed to combat anxious feelings throughout the day.

4. Keep the roll-on in a cool, dark place between applications.

Tip: Use any blend of anti-anxiety essential oils to create a similar roll-on. Experiment with scents to create a personalized solution.

Bad Breath

Some of the best foods for our health (garlic, anyone?) leave behind quite a pungent smell. Bad breath can sometimes accompany illnesses, too; if you're not sure why you have halitosis, check with your doctor to determine the cause.

Helpful Essential Oils: clove, lavender, lemon, lemongrass, peppermint, thyme

PEPPERMINT BREATH SPRAY

TOPICAL, SAFE FOR CHILDREN AGES 12+

MUST HAVE You don't have to chew gum to enjoy minty-fresh breath! This quick, easy spray is portable, plus it's sweetened with stevia, an all-natural, zero-calorie sweetener. MAKES ABOUT ¼ CUP

¼ cup distilled water
5 drops peppermint essential oil

3 drops liquid stevia

1. In a small glass bottle fitted with a spray top, combine the distilled water, peppermint essential oil, and stevia. Cap the bottle and shake well to blend. Shake again before each use.

2. Apply 1 or 2 spritzes to the inside of your mouth anytime you feel not so fresh. Repeat as needed.

3. Keep your breath spray in a cool, dark place between uses.

Tip: Don't like peppermint? Try a different oil.

LEMON-CLOVE BREATH DROPS

TOPICAL, SAFE FOR CHILDREN AGES 12+

MUST HAVE Quick and easy to make, this blend contains lemon and clove, two essential oils that kill the bacteria responsible for bad breath. Packaged in a tiny bottle, it's portable for on-the-go freshening. MAKES ABOUT 50 TREATMENTS

1½ teaspoons vodka
1 drop clove essential oil

1 drop lemon essential oil
1 drop liquid stevia

1. In a small glass bottle with an orifice reducer or medicine dropper top, combine the vodka, clove, and lemon essential oils, and stevia. Cap the bottle and shake well to blend. Shake again before each use.

2. Apply 1 drop of the blend to the underside of your tongue for fresher breath. Repeat as needed.

3. Keep your breath drops in a cool, dry place between uses.

   Tip: Vodka kills germs just like essential oils; however, you can use water for an alcohol-free version.

Body Odor

Commercial products designed to eliminate body odor can contain potentially harmful ingredients, plus they can be expensive. Natural deodorants made with essential oils won't keep you from sweating, but they do kill bacteria that cause body odor, while being easy on your pocketbook.

Helpful Essential Oils: clary sage, frankincense, geranium, lavender, lemongrass, patchouli, peppermint, rosemary, tea tree, thyme

LEMONGRASS DEODORANT

TOPICAL, SAFE FOR CHILDREN AGES 12+

MUST HAVE Lemongrass is such an effective deodorizer that it's a top ingredient in some bestselling natural deodorant brands. This solution is great for preventing foot odor, too. MAKES ABOUT ½ CUP

30 drops lemongrass essential oil
¼ cup coconut oil

¼ cup tapioca flour, or arrowroot powder

1. In a small bowl, blend together the lemongrass essential oil, coconut oil, and tapioca flour with a spoon or spatula until the consistency resembles thick toothpaste. Transfer the deodorant to a shallow jar with a tight-fitting lid.

2. With your fingertips, apply a pea-size amount of deodorant to each underarm, using a little more or less as needed. Give the deodorant a minute or two to absorb into your skin before getting dressed. If you're wearing a dark-colored top, you might want to dress before applying the deodorant; otherwise, it may leave streaks. Repeat once or twice daily as needed.

3. Keep your deodorant in a cool, dry place between uses.

Tip: You may want to keep this remedy refrigerated during hot weather. If it gets too warm, the ingredients may separate. If this occurs, just reblend and continue using.

LAVENDER-LEMONGRASS DEODORANT SPRAY

TOPICAL, SAFE FOR CHILDREN AGES 12+

MUST HAVE Lavender and lemongrass essential oils blend with witch hazel and magnesium oil and a pinch of natural sea salt, killing bacteria and reducing body odor, while preventing any unsightly streaks on clothing. Note that magnesium oil can be hard on sensitive skin, so you may want to omit it if your skin is more delicate. MAKES ABOUT ½ CUP

30 drops lavender essential oil

30 drops lemongrass essential oil

⅛ teaspoon unprocessed sea salt, or fine Himalayan salt

6 tablespoons alcohol-free witch hazel

1½ tablespoons magnesium oil (optional)

1. In a glass bottle fitted with a spray top, combine the lavender and lemongrass essential oils. Let them rest for at least 1 hour.

2. Add the salt and swirl to combine.

3. Add the witch hazel and magnesium oil (if using), cap the bottle, and shake well to combine. Shake again before each use.

4. Apply 1 to 2 spritzes to each underarm. Repeat as needed.

5. Keep the deodorant in a cool, dry place between uses.

Tip: You can easily make your own signature deodorant by substituting your favorite essential oils for the ones called for here.

Chapped Lips

Cold weather and dry indoor air often lead to chapped lips. Aromatherapy balms help your lips heal, while eliminating the risks that come with overexposure to petroleum products in many commercial solutions.

Helpful Essential Oils: clary sage, eucalyptus, frankincense, geranium, lavender, patchouli, Roman chamomile, tea tree

SOOTHING ROMAN CHAMOMILE LIP BALM

TOPICAL, SAFE FOR CHILDREN AGES 2+

This rich, moisturizing balm takes some effort to make, but you'll love the results. Roman chamomile soothes chapped lips and promotes faster healing, as do honey, beeswax, and coconut oil. This recipe makes enough to fill about four empty lip balm tubes.

MAKES 4 LIP BALMS

4 teaspoons coconut oil

2 teaspoons beeswax pastilles, or grated beeswax

6 drops vitamin E oil (optional)

½ teaspoon honey (optional)

4 drops Roman chamomile essential oil

1. In a small glass bowl, combine the coconut oil, beeswax, vitamin E oil (if using), and honey (if using). Cover the bowl and microwave on low power for 5 seconds. Stir, re-cover the bowl, and microwave for 5 seconds more. If you don't have a microwave, melt the ingredients in a clean, dry double boiler over low heat.

2. Stir in the Roman chamomile essential oil. Quickly transfer the blend to 4 clean, dry lip balm tubes, or small jars with tight-fitting lids. Let the lip balm cool completely before you cap it to prevent condensation from forming.

3. Apply the balm to lips as needed throughout the day.

4. Keep your balm in a convenient location where it won't be exposed to heat.

Tip: If you prefer a vegan option, or want to use the balm for a child too young for bee products, replace the honey and beeswax with carnauba wax or candelilla wax.

QUICK LAVENDER-MINT LIP BALM

TOPICAL, SAFE FOR CHILDREN AGES 2+

MUST HAVE If you need a quick fix, you'll appreciate this ultra-simple lip balm, which contains lavender essential oil to help heal any chapping, plus peppermint for a refreshing feel. It's easiest to package this in a roller bottle, but you can use a small, dark-colored glass bottle if you prefer. MAKES ABOUT 1 TABLESPOON

4 drops lavender essential oil
1 drop peppermint essential oil

1 tablespoon fractionated coconut oil

1. In a roller bottle, combine the lavender and peppermint essential oils and fractionated coconut oil. Cap the bottle and shake well to combine.

2. Dab 1 or 2 drops onto your lips. Either press your lips together or use your fingertip to spread the balm, just don't overdo it. Repeat as needed.

3. Keep your balm in a convenient location away from heat.

Tip: If lips are extremely chapped, consider omitting the peppermint essential oil and increasing the lavender to 6 drops. The scent will be stronger, and so will the healing effect.

AROMATHERAPY FOR BEGINNERS

Combination Skin Care

Dry cheeks, an oily T-zone, or some other combination? Combination skin can be tricky to care for, and products can be expensive. Aromatherapy offers a variety of solutions for balancing combination skin without damaging your budget.

Helpful Essential Oils: clary sage, eucalyptus, frankincense, geranium, grapefruit, lavender, lemon, lemongrass, patchouli, Roman chamomile, tea tree

PATCHOULI-ROMAN CHAMOMILE SUGAR SCRUB

TOPICAL, SAFE FOR CHILDREN AGES 12+

Cleanse and exfoliate in one quick step with this comforting sugar scrub. Patchouli and Roman chamomile essential oils nourish and balance skin, and add a lovely scent to your daily routine.
MAKES ABOUT 1 CUP

8 drops patchouli essential oil	½ cup sweet almond oil
4 drops Roman chamomile essential oil	½ cup sugar

1. In a jar with a tight-fitting lid, combine the patchouli and Roman chamomile essential oils. Let the blend rest for at least 1 hour.

2. Using a thin utensil, such as a fork or butter knife, stir in the almond oil and sugar to blend completely.

3. Dampen your face with warm water. With your fingertips, apply about ½ teaspoon of the sugar scrub. Using gentle circular motions, cleanse your entire face.

4. Rinse with warm water, and pat dry. Repeat daily.

5. Keep the scrub in a convenient location away from heat.

   Tip: Try it in the shower to smooth and moisturize your body!

BALANCING CLARY SAGE-TEA TREE MOISTURIZER

TOPICAL, SAFE FOR CHILDREN AGES 12+

Clary sage and tea tree address occasional breakouts, while coconut oil and vitamin E offer quick-absorbing moisture. This simple treatment is ideal for your face, neck, and chest, plus you can use it to treat dry knees, elbows, heels, and more. MAKES ABOUT ¼ CUP

3 drops clary sage essential oil

3 drops tea tree essential oil

½ teaspoon vitamin E oil

¼ cup coconut oil

1. In a small jar with a tight-fitting lid, combine the clary sage and tea tree essential oils. Let them rest for at least 1 hour.

2. With a thin utensil, such as a chopstick, stir in the vitamin E and coconut oils until all ingredients are well combined.

3. With your fingertip, apply a pea-size amount of moisturizer to your face, using a little more or less as needed. Repeat morning and evening for best results.

4. Store your moisturizer in a cool, dark place between uses.

Tip: You can create a customized moisturizer with any blend or single essential oil that meets your needs. Try lavender, Roman chamomile, or lemongrass.

Dandruff

You're not alone if dandruff is an issue; many people experience a dry, flaky scalp at times. Because dandruff is often caused or exacerbated by fungus, antifungal essential oils tend to work best. These oils also soothe itching and help irritated skin heal, returning your scalp to a healthy state.

Helpful Essential Oils: clary sage, clove, eucalyptus, lavender, lemongrass, patchouli, Roman chamomile, rosemary, tea tree, thyme

ROSEMARY–TEA TREE SHAMPOO

TOPICAL, SAFE FOR CHILDREN AGES 2+

MUST HAVE Fragrance-free shampoo combines with refreshing rosemary and tea tree essential oils, letting you lather up as usual, while enjoying a pleasant aromatherapy experience. This shampoo is mild enough to use every day, either to treat or prevent dandruff. MAKES ABOUT 1 CUP

30 drops rosemary essential oil   1 cup fragrance-free shampoo

15 drops tea tree essential oil

1. In a small glass bottle with a tight-fitting lid, combine the rosemary and tea tree essential oils. Let them rest for at least 1 hour.

2. In a small bowl, combine the shampoo with the blended essential oils. Using a whisk or handheld mixer, blend thoroughly. Use a funnel to carefully transfer the finished product to an 8-ounce bottle.

3. Use about 1 teaspoon of shampoo to wash your hair while bathing or showering, applying a little more or less as needed. Lather well and let the shampoo sit on your scalp for at least 30 seconds before rinsing. Repeat if your hair tends to be oily, and follow up with conditioner such as Lemongrass Conditioner (page 166). Let your hair air-dry, if possible, as hot air from a blow dryer can aggravate dandruff.

4. Keep your shampoo in a convenient location away from heat.

Tip: This blend has a refreshing scent, but some people find it medicinal. Consider adding 10 to 20 drops of lavender essential oil to soften the fragrance.

TOPICAL, SAFE FOR CHILDREN AGES 2+

MUST HAVE Lemongrass essential oil is an outstanding antifungal agent, and its pleasant, refreshing scent lifts your spirits. Fragrance-free conditioner makes it simple to give your hair customized care, while helping your scalp return to a smooth, flake-free state. MAKES ABOUT 1 CUP

1 cup fragrance-free conditioner   40 drops lemongrass essential oil

1. In a small bowl, combine the conditioner with the lemongrass essential oil. Using a whisk or handheld mixer, blend thoroughly. Use a funnel to carefully transfer the finished product to an 8-ounce bottle.

2. Use about 1 teaspoon of conditioner after shampooing, allowing it to sit on your scalp for at least 30 seconds before rinsing. Let your hair air-dry, if possible, as hot air from a blow dryer can aggravate dandruff.

3. Keep your conditioner in a convenient location away from heat.

Tip: No lemongrass? Use an equal amount of lavender or eucalyptus essential oil, or try 20 drops of clove essential oil.

Depression

Whether you have an unexplainable case of the blues or have been diagnosed with clinical depression, aromatherapy may help you manage your symptoms. Talk to your doctor about adding essential oils to your routine if you take medications for your depression, and do not reduce your dose or stop taking prescriptions without your doctor's approval.

Helpful Essential Oils: clary sage, frankincense, geranium, grapefruit, lavender, lemon, patchouli, peppermint, Roman chamomile, rosemary

EASY LAVENDER MASSAGE

TOPICAL, SAFE FOR CHILDREN AGES 12+

MUST HAVE Lavender's uplifting effect is legendary, and there's some solid science to uphold anecdotes about its antidepressant effect. Studies have shown that lavender essential oil reduces depression and related issues including postpartum depression, anxiety, and stress. MAKES ABOUT 1 TABLESPOON

24 drops lavender essential oil

1 tablespoon fractionated coconut oil

1. In a roller bottle, combine the lavender essential oil and fractionated coconut oil. Cap the bottle and shake well to combine.

2. Dab a bit of the blend behind each ear. Repeat as often as you like, particularly when you have time to relax or engage in an enjoyable activity.

3. Keep the roll-on in a cool, dark place between applications.

Tip: If you don't have time to make this roll-on, simply diffuse lavender or apply a few drops of essential oil to your clothing. You'll receive aromatherapy benefits without much effort.

UPLIFTING DIFFUSER BLEND

AROMATIC, SAFE FOR ALL AGES

Clary sage, frankincense, grapefruit, and lavender essential oils deliver an intoxicating scent and lift your spirits. This wonderful blend can be used in aromatherapy jewelry or essential oil inhalers, or added to bath products. MAKES ABOUT 30 TREATMENTS

20 drops clary sage essential oil
20 drops frankincense essential oil

30 drops grapefruit essential oil
30 drops lavender essential oil

1. In a dark-colored glass bottle with a dropper or orifice reducer, combine the clary sage, frankincense, grapefruit, and lavender essential oils. Let them rest for at least 1 hour.

2. Add 3 or 4 drops of the blend to a diffuser and use according to the manufacturer's instructions. Repeat any time anxious thoughts intrude.

3. Keep your diffuser blend in a cool, dark place between uses.

   Tip: If you like this blend, add it to a roller bottle. Just combine 8 to 10 drops of the blend with 1 tablespoon fractionated coconut oil, and apply it to pulse points when you need an emotional boost.

Dry Skin Care

Dry skin can be irritatingly itchy. The good news is, aromatherapy products made with rich emollients and balancing essential oils can reduce itching and flakiness, while increasing softness and imparting a healthier appearance. Use them regularly and enjoy the results.

Helpful Essential Oils: clary sage, frankincense, geranium, lavender, patchouli, Roman chamomile, rosemary

BALANCING GERANIUM MOISTURIZER

TOPICAL, SAFE FOR CHILDREN AGES 2+

MUST HAVE Geranium essential oil balances and tones skin, plus it promotes elasticity by increasing natural oil production when needed. Coconut oil contributes lasting moisture and provides a barrier between dry skin and harsh elements.

MAKES ABOUT ½ CUP

32 drops geranium essential oil
½ cup coconut oil, barely melted

1. In a jar with a tight-fitting lid, combine the geranium essential oil and coconut oil. Using a thin utensil, such as a chopstick, blend completely.

2. With your fingertips, apply a pea-size amount of the blend to each area of dry skin, using a little more or less as needed. Repeat as often as you like, particularly after bathing and showering, before bed, and a few minutes before getting dressed each day.

3. Keep your moisturizer in a cool, dark place between uses.

Tip: If you don't want to use coconut oil every day, add geranium essential oil to your favorite fragrance-free body lotion: 32 drops of essential oil to ½ cup of body lotion.

ROMAN CHAMOMILE-FRANKINCENSE FACIAL MOISTURIZER

TOPICAL, SAFE FOR ALL AGES

MUST HAVE Roman chamomile and frankincense essential oils are gentle on inflamed, itchy skin, while apricot kernel, rosehip, and coconut oils combine with cocoa butter and vegetable glycerin to offer lasting moisture. MAKES ABOUT 1 CUP

10 drops frankincense essential oil

15 drops Roman chamomile essential oil

½ cup cocoa butter

½ cup coconut oil

1½ teaspoons apricot kernel oil

1½ teaspoons rosehip oil (optional)

1 tablespoon vegetable glycerin (optional)

1. In a dark-colored glass bottle with a tight-fitting lid, combine the frankincense and Roman chamomile essential oils. Let them rest overnight.

2. In the clean, dry bowl of a blender or food processor, combine the essential oil blend, cocoa butter, coconut oil, apricot kernel

oil, and rosehip oil and glycerin (if using). Process until smooth. Transfer the blend to a clean, dry bowl, and refrigerate until firm.

3. With the whip or whisk attachment of a stand mixer or with a handheld electric mixer, process the blend until it has a light, silky texture. Transfer the finished cream to a jar with a tight-fitting lid.

4. After washing your face, use your fingers to apply a pea-size amount of the moisturizer, using a little more or less as needed. Repeat once or twice daily.

5. Keep your moisturizer in a cool, dark place between uses.

Tip: Out of frankincense? Try blending Roman chamomile with any essential oil recommended for dry skin. Its mild fragrance makes it a versatile choice for creating your own blends.

Emotional Upset

Aromatherapy can help you cope a little better with life's sad, angry, upsetting events by supporting healthy cognition, balancing emotions, and giving your mood a much-needed boost. Although essential oils won't stop you from experiencing unpleasantness, they can make it easier to manage life's hiccups.

Helpful Essential Oils: clary sage, clove, frankincense, grapefruit, lemon, lemongrass, patchouli, peppermint, Roman chamomile, rosemary

LEMON-GRAPEFRUIT DIFFUSER BLEND

AROMATIC, SAFE FOR ALL AGES

Lemon and grapefruit essential oils mingle here to boost even the bluest mood, while awakening the senses. This simple blend can be used in aromatherapy jewelry or essential oil inhalers, and it can be added to bath products, as long as you follow precautions regarding exposure to sunlight. MAKES ABOUT 20 TREATMENTS

30 drops grapefruit essential oil   30 drops lemon essential oil

1. In a dark-colored glass bottle with a dropper or orifice reducer, combine the grapefruit and lemon essential oils. Let them rest for at least 1 hour.

2. Add 3 or 4 drops of the blend to a diffuser and use according to the manufacturer's instructions. Repeat any time you need cheering up.

3. Keep your diffuser blend in a cool, dark place between uses.

Tip: If you decide to expand your aromatherapy repertoire, consider adding other citrus oils to this blend. Bergamot, lime, and mandarin are some wonderful ones to try.

FRANKINCENSE ROLL-ON

TOPICAL, SAFE FOR CHILDREN AGES 12+

MUST HAVE Frankincense helps ground unpleasant emotions and can promote a sense of peaceful calm. This simple roll-on is particularly helpful when you're feeling cranky, overwhelmed, or downright angry. MAKES ABOUT 1 TABLESPOON

18 drops frankincense   1 tablespoon fractionated
essential oil   coconut oil

1. In a roller bottle, combine the frankincense essential oil and fractionated coconut oil. Cap the bottle and shake well to combine.

2. Swipe the roller across your wrists. Use your fingertips to rub the blend into your hands, inhaling deeply, while focusing on happier times ahead. Repeat as needed to combat negativity of all kinds.

3. Keep the roll-on in a cool, dark place between applications.

Tip: If you want to use frankincense to calm children under 12 years, use 8 drops of essential oil to formulate a special that is safe for them.

Exhaustion

When you find yourself overwhelmed physically and/or mentally, let aromatherapy come to the rescue. Try calming essential oils if you're in a position to rest and relax; choose uplifting ones if you need to keep on going. Aromatherapy inhalers are ideal for keeping your favorite singles and blends nearby, particularly when you're on the go.

Helpful Essential Oils: clary sage, frankincense, geranium, grapefruit, lavender, lemon, lemongrass, patchouli, Roman chamomile, rosemary

UPLIFTING CITRUS-ROSEMARY DIFFUSER BLEND

AROMATIC, SAFE FOR ALL AGES

Lemon and grapefruit essential oils soften rosemary's sharp scent, while waking you up a bit so you can keep on with your day. This simple blend can be used in aromatherapy jewelry or essential oil inhalers, and it can be added to bath products, as long as you follow precautions regarding exposure to sunlight.

MAKES ABOUT 30 TREATMENTS

30 drops grapefruit essential oil   30 drops rosemary essential oil

30 drops lemon essential oil

1. In a dark-colored glass bottle with a dropper or orifice reducer, combine the grapefruit, lemon, and rosemary essential oils. Let them rest for at least 1 hour before using.

2. Add 3 or 4 drops of the blend to a diffuser and use according to the manufacturer's instructions. Repeat any time you need cheering up.

3. Keep your diffuser blend in a cool, dark place between uses.

Tip: No rosemary? Try peppermint essential oil in its place.

RELAXING ROMAN CHAMOMILE-PATCHOULI ROLL-ON

TOPICAL, SAFE FOR CHILDREN AGES 12+

When you've put in a long day and are ready for some down time, Roman chamomile and patchouli essential oils can help you relax without making you sleepy. This roll-on is just right for transitioning from work to more pleasant activities. MAKES ABOUT 1 TABLESPOON

6 drops patchouli essential oil

12 drops Roman chamomile essential oil

1 tablespoon fractionated coconut oil

1. In a roller bottle, combine the patchouli and Roman chamomile essential oils with the fractionated coconut oil. Cap the bottle and shake well to combine.

2. Swipe the roller across your wrists. Use your fingertips to rub the blend into your hands, inhaling deeply. Take a few minutes to relax, if possible. Repeat as needed.

3. Keep the roll-on in a cool, dark place between applications.

Tip: Not a fan of patchouli? Try frankincense essential oil instead, or enjoy Roman chamomile essential oil on its own.

Hair Health

Shiny, healthy hair doesn't have to be hard to achieve, but conventional products often contain unwanted chemicals and come at higher prices than you might want to pay. Try aromatherapy next time you're looking for a good way to improve your hair's look and feel. It's surprisingly easy to create your own blends that leave your hair soft, shiny, and manageable.

Helpful Essential Oils: clary sage, clove, eucalyptus, geranium, grapefruit, lavender, lemon, lemongrass, patchouli, peppermint, Roman chamomile, rosemary, tea tree, thyme

BALANCING SHAMPOO

TOPICAL, SAFE FOR CHILDREN AGES 2+

MUST HAVE Soothing lavender and crisp peppermint mingle with irresistible rosemary for a delightful scent that transforms your shower into a mini spa experience. This shampoo is mild enough to use every day, and takes just a little time to formulate.
MAKES ABOUT 1 CUP

20 drops lavender essential oil	3 drops rosemary essential oil
5 drops peppermint essential oil	1 cup fragrance-free shampoo

1. In a small glass bottle with a tight-fitting lid, combine the lavender, peppermint, and rosemary essential oils. Let them rest for at least 1 hour.

2. In a small bowl, combine the shampoo with the essential oils blend. Using a whisk or handheld mixer, blend thoroughly. Use a funnel to carefully transfer the finished product to an 8-ounce bottle.

3. Use about 1 teaspoon of shampoo to wash your hair while bathing or showering, applying a little more or less as needed. Lather well and let the shampoo sit on your scalp for at least

30 seconds before rinsing. Repeat if your hair tends to be oily, and follow up with a conditioner, such as Lemongrass Leave-In Conditioner (below). Let your hair air-dry, if possible, as hot air from a blow dryer can aggravate dandruff.

4. Keep your shampoo in a convenient place where it won't be exposed to high temperatures.

Tip: This blend is easy to customize. If you're not sure how your chosen scents will smell, make a mini-batch with 2 tablespoons of shampoo or less. Play with the amounts and types of oil you use to create your personal favorite.

LEMONGRASS LEAVE-IN CONDITIONER

TOPICAL, SAFE FOR CHILDREN AGES 2+

MUST HAVE Lemongrass helps keep your scalp healthy, plus its fragrance is refreshing. With this simple leave-in treatment, a little fragrance-free conditioner and a few drops of essential oil go a long way toward keeping your hair soft and manageable.

MAKES ABOUT 1 CUP

1 cup distilled water
2 tablespoons fragrance-free
    conditioner

16 drops lemongrass essential oil

1. In a bottle fitted with a spray top, combine the distilled water, conditioner, and lemongrass essential oil. Cap the bottle and shake well to blend completely. Shake again briefly before each use.

2. After shampooing and towel-drying your hair, apply just enough conditioner to cover it. Brush or comb the conditioner through, and style your hair as usual.

Tip: If your hair tends to be dry or frizzy, use a quick spritz even when hair is dry to get things under control.

Oily Hair

If you have oily hair, your natural inclination might be to wash it repeatedly with harsh shampoos that strip away all the oil. The short-term results might be alright, but your scalp goes into over-drive, producing more oil to replace what was lost. Balancing, clarifying essential oils help keep your hair looking its best.

Helpful Essential Oils: clary sage, clove, eucalyptus, geranium, grapefruit, lavender, lemon, lemongrass, patchouli, Roman chamomile, rosemary, tea tree, thyme

LEMON-THYME RINSE

TOPICAL, SAFE FOR CHILDREN AGES 6+

Lemon and thyme essential oils pair with apple cider vinegar, decreasing residue on your scalp, unclogging hair follicles, and imparting incredible body and shine. Natural, nonpasteurized apple cider vinegar with "the mother" works best, but you can use pasteurized, or white vinegar, in a pinch. MAKES ABOUT 8 TREATMENTS

1 cup apple cider vinegar
6 drops lemon essential oil
4 drops thyme essential oil

1. In a bottle or jar, combine the cider vinegar and lemon and thyme essential oils. Let the blend rest for at least 24 hours before using it, and keep it in a cool, dark place between uses.

2. In a plastic squeeze bottle, mix 2 tablespoons of the rinse with 1 cup of water.

3. Shampoo your hair as usual and rinse it with plain water to remove the suds. Apply the entire squeeze bottle of the rinse to your hair, and leave it in for at least 30 seconds.

4. Rinse with water, towel-dry, and style your hair as usual. Repeat the treatment 3 to 4 times weekly.

5. Keep your rinse in a cool, dark place between uses.

   Tip: If you like, leave the rinse in your hair, squeeze out the excess, towel-dry, and style. Using the blend as a leave-in provides additional conditioning benefits.

TEA TREE DRY SHAMPOO

TOPICAL, SAFE FOR CHILDREN AGES 6+

MUST HAVE Dry shampoo absorbs oil from your scalp without completely stripping moisture, and tea tree essential oil prevents bacterial buildup that can lead to dandruff and itching. If you have light-colored hair, use cornstarch; if you have dark hair, use cinnamon. MAKES ABOUT ½ CUP

5 drops tea tree essential oil	½ cup cornstarch, or
	½ cup ground cinnamon

1. In a jar with a tight-fitting lid, combine the tea tree essential oil with the cornstarch or cinnamon. Cover the container and shake to blend thoroughly.

2. With a cosmetics brush (a blush-size brush is ideal), apply a light coating of dry shampoo to the roots of your hair. Use just enough to cover oily areas.

3. With your fingertips, lightly massage your scalp. Wait about 30 seconds, and brush or comb your hair to remove any excess powder. Style your hair as usual.

4. Keep your dry shampoo in a cool, dry place between uses.

   Tip: If you like using dry shampoo, try this strategy: Use regular shampoo in the shower on day one, skip shampooing on day two (rinse your head with plain water in the shower), and use dry shampoo on day three. On day four, re-start the cycle with regular shampoo.

Oily Skin Care

Your skin's natural oils provide protection from the elements and hold moisture in, but excess oil gives your face a shiny look, and can contribute to acne. Many cleansers strip too much moisture from skin and compound the problem by causing oil production to increase. Try these treatments next time you want balanced skin.

Helpful Essential Oils: clary sage, clove, eucalyptus, geranium, grapefruit, lavender, lemon, lemongrass, patchouli, Roman chamomile, rosemary, tea tree, thyme

LAVENDER OATMEAL MASK

TOPICAL, SAFE FOR CHILDREN AGES 6+

MUST HAVE Soothing oatmeal and lavender essential oils work to absorb excess oil without drying skin. This treatment takes just a few minutes, and it leaves your skin feeling soft and smooth.

MAKES 1 TREATMENT

¼ cup dry instant oatmeal	1 teaspoon water
2 teaspoons freshly squeezed lemon juice	2 drops lavender essential oil

1. In a bowl, combine the oatmeal, lemon juice, water, and lavender essential oil. Using a fork, stir until a thick paste forms.

2. Wet your face and use your fingers to apply the mask. Let the mask dry, and rinse it off with water. Repeat 2 to 3 times weekly, or whenever oily skin is a problem.

Tip: If you have blackheads, whiteheads, or pimples, try tea tree essential oil instead of lavender.

ROMAN CHAMOMILE–TEA TREE TONER

TOPICAL, SAFE FOR CHILDREN AGES 12+

Tea tree, Roman chamomile, and green tea blend with witch hazel, breaking up excess oil without stripping skin. When used daily, this toner can help prevent breakouts. MAKES ABOUT ½ CUP

3 drops Roman chamomile essential oil

3 drops tea tree essential oil

1 green tea bag

¼ cup steaming-hot water

3 tablespoons alcohol-free witch hazel

1 teaspoon freshly squeezed lemon juice

1 teaspoon baking soda

1. In a 4-ounce bottle with a tight-fitting top, combine the Roman chamomile and tea tree essential oils. Let them rest for at least 1 hour.

2. In a liquid measuring cup, steep the teabag in the hot water until the water cools. Remove and discard the teabag.

3. Stir the witch hazel, lemon juice, and baking soda into the tea, stirring until the baking soda dissolves completely. Using a funnel to prevent spills, transfer the liquid mixture to the bottle with the blended essential oils.

4. With a cotton ball or cosmetic pad, apply about ¼ teaspoon of toner to your freshly washed face. Repeat once or twice daily.

5. Refrigerate, where your toner will stay fresh for up to 8 weeks.

Tip: If you think you'll use more than ½ cup during an 8-week period, consider making a double batch.

Scars

While scars can be a visceral reminder of challenges you've over-come, you may want to prevent them or at least reduce their appearance. Commercial products are effective, but often expensive. Aromatherapy treatments can be just as helpful, and are far easier on your budget.

Helpful Essential Oils: clary sage, frankincense, geranium, lavender, patchouli, Roman chamomile, tea tree

FRANKINCENSE-TEA TREE FADING BALM

TOPICAL, SAFE FOR CHILDREN AGES 6+

MUST HAVE Tea tree and frankincense essential oils help wounds heal faster and help scars fade. The sooner you use this balm, the better your results are likely to be. MAKES ABOUT ¼ CUP

8 drops frankincense essential oil   ¼ cup coconut oil, barely melted
3 drops tea tree essential oil

1. In a jar with a tight-fitting lid, combine the frankincense and tea tree essential oils. Let them rest for at least 1 hour before proceeding.

2. Using a thin utensil, such as a chopstick, stir in the coconut oil until blended completely.

3. With your fingertips or a cotton swab, apply a drop of balm to the scar, using a little more or less as needed. Repeat at least twice daily, and don't lose hope. It can take several weeks to see results.

4. Keep the balm in a cool, dark place between uses.

Tip: If the treated area won't be exposed to sunlight, you can add 4 drops of lemon essential oil to this blend. It contains high levels of vitamin C, which helps skin heal faster.

GERANIUM SCAR TONER

TOPICAL, SAFE FOR CHILDREN AGES 6+

MUST HAVE Geranium essential oil is a powerful cicatrizant, meaning it promotes healing and cell regeneration. Apple cider vinegar helps remove dead skin cells and fade dark spots, making this combination a good one to try on old scars. While this toner may not remove your scars completely, it's likely to reduce angry red and purple colors, especially when skin is actively healing.

MAKES ABOUT ¼ CUP

48 drops geranium essential oil   ¼ cup apple cider vinegar

1. In a bottle or jar with a tight-fitting lid, combine the geranium essential oil and cider vinegar. Cover the container and shake well to blend. Shake again before each use.

2. With a cotton ball or cosmetic pad, apply about ¼ teaspoon of the toner to the scarred area, using a little more or less as needed. Repeat once or twice daily until desired results are obtained.

3. Keep the toner in a cool, dark place between uses.

   Tip: No geranium essential oil? Formulate a similar toner with any essential oil recommended for treating scars.

Spider Veins

Visible blood vessels that look blue, purple, or dark red can be eliminated via sclerotherapy or laser surgery, however these treatments can be expensive and can sometimes produce permanent changes in skin color. Aromatherapy can help reduce the appearance of spider veins, particularly if used in conjunction with supportive therapies, such as exercise or massage.

Helpful Essential Oils: clary sage, eucalyptus, frankincense, geranium, grapefruit, lemon, peppermint, Roman chamomile, rosemary

CLARY SAGE–GERANIUM MASSAGE

TOPICAL, SAFE FOR AGES 12+

Clary sage and geranium essential oils promote healing and improve circulation, while sunflower oil offers anti-inflammatory benefits. As with many therapies, this simple massage works best when used frequently and consistently. MAKES ABOUT ¼ CUP

20 drops clary sage essential oil   ¼ cup sunflower oil
10 drops geranium essential oil

1. In a bottle with a tight-fitting lid, combine the clary sage and geranium essential oils. Let them rest for at least 1 hour.

2. Add the sunflower oil to the bottle, cap it, and shake well to combine.

3. With your fingertips, apply about ½ teaspoon of the blend to the affected area and massage with slow, firm strokes in the direction of the heart. Repeat the massage at least twice daily.

4. Keep the massage oil in a cool, dark place between treatments.

Tip: Consider massaging right after you wake up and again just before you go to sleep. If you can, consider adding a third treatment when you can elevate your legs for 20 to 30 minutes.

SYNERGISTIC SPIDER VEIN CREAM

TOPICAL, MAY CAUSE PHOTOSENSITIVITY, SAFE FOR AGES 12+

This cream promotes better circulation, which in turn can strengthen blood vessel walls and reduce the appearance of spider veins. The mango butter, coconut oil, and jojoba oil provide moisture, improving the overall appearance of skin. If you don't have mango butter, substitute shea or cocoa butter. MAKES ABOUT 1 CUP

10 drops geranium essential oil

20 drops lemon essential oil

10 drops Roman chamomile
essential oil

10 drops rosemary essential oil

½ cup mango butter

¼ cup coconut oil

¼ cup jojoba oil

1. In a small bottle, combine the geranium, lemon, Roman chamomile, and rosemary essential oils. Let them rest overnight, if possible, but at least 1 hour.

2. In a double boiler over medium-low heat, combine the mango butter and coconut oil. Stir until the ingredients are just melted.

3. Add the jojoba oil and the blended essential oils. Stir to combine. Transfer the liquefied blend to a small bowl and refrigerate for 2 hours.

4. With a handheld mixer, whip the solidified cream until it has a light silky, texture. Transfer it to a jar with a tight-fitting lid.

5. Use your fingertips to apply ½ teaspoon of the body cream to each affected area, massaging with firm strokes in the direction of your heart. Repeat at least twice daily.

6. Store your cream in a cool, dark place between uses.

Tip: This cream will melt if it gets too warm. You can restore its texture by chilling and whipping it again.

Stretch Marks

Stretch marks are small scars that start as angry-looking red or purple stripes, which eventually fade to a silver or white color. While it's impossible to prevent or remove them completely, aromatherapy treatments can often reduce their appearance and improve skin's texture.

Helpful Essential Oils: clary sage, frankincense, geranium, lavender, patchouli, Roman chamomile, tea tree

SYNERGISTIC STRETCH MARK BALM

TOPICAL, SAFE FOR AGES 12+

This cream promotes healing, and it can reduce the appearance of stretch marks. The cocoa butter, coconut oil, and jojoba oil provide deep moisture. Don't be surprised if you find yourself applying this lovely moisturizer even to unaffected areas! MAKES ABOUT 1 CUP

10 drops geranium essential oil
20 drops lavender essential oil
10 drops patchouli essential oil
10 drops Roman chamomile
    essential oil

½ cup cocoa butter
¼ cup coconut oil
¼ cup jojoba oil

1. In a small bottle, combine the geranium, lavender, patchouli, and Roman chamomile essential oils. Let them rest overnight.

2. In a double boiler over medium-low heat, combine the cocoa butter and coconut oil. Stir until the ingredients are just melted.

3. Add the jojoba oil and the blended essential oils. Transfer the liquefied blend to a small bowl and refrigerate for 2 hours.

4. With a handheld mixer, whip the solidified cream until it has a light, silky texture. Transfer the balm to a jar with a tight-fitting lid.

5. Use your fingertips to apply ½ teaspoon of the cream to each affected area and repeat at least twice daily.

6. Store the cream in a cool, dark place between uses.

   Tip: You can use mango or shea butter instead of the cocoa butter, or leave out the jojoba oil and cocoa butter in favor of a simpler balm made with 1 cup coconut oil.

LAVENDER-SESAME MASSAGE

TOPICAL, SAFE FOR ALL AGES

MUST HAVE Lavender is known for its ability to fade scars, including stretch marks, and sesame oil offers healing and nourishing properties of its own. This simple remedy works best when applied to new stretch marks. MAKES ABOUT ½ CUP

32 drops lavender essential oil ½ cup sesame oil

1. In a bottle with a tight-fitting lid, combine the lavender essential oil and sesame oil. Cap the bottle and shake well to combine.

2. With your fingertips, apply about ¼ teaspoon of the massage oil to each affected area, using a little bit more or less as needed. Gently massage, and give the oil time to absorb into your skin before dressing. Repeat at least twice daily.

3. Keep your massage oil in a cool, dark place between uses.

Tip: If you don't love the smell of sesame oil, make this blend with shea butter instead. It's another good carrier for stretch mark-fighting blends.

Stress

Stress feels terrible, and too much can damage your health. It's impossible to avoid stressful circumstances completely, but you can use aromatherapy as a strategy for taking mini vacations and rebalancing your mind. Most essential oils can help improve your mental state; it's a good idea to experiment and find out what feels best to you.

Helpful Essential Oils: clary sage, clove, frankincense, grapefruit, lavender, lemon, lemongrass, patchouli, Roman chamomile, rosemary, thyme

RELAXING DIFFUSER BLEND

AROMATIC, SAFE FOR ALL AGES

Lemon, lavender, and clary sage essential oils balance one another perfectly, while promoting a cheerful atmosphere. This blend is just right for diffusing after work, when you're ready to relax and enjoy the evening. MAKES ABOUT 30 TREATMENTS

30 drops clary sage essential oil

30 drops lavender essential oil

30 drops lemon essential oil

1. In a dark-colored glass bottle with a dropper or orifice reducer, combine the clary sage, lavender, and lemon essential oils. Let them rest for at least 1 hour.

2. Add 3 or 4 drops of the blend to a diffuser and use according to the manufacturer's instructions. Repeat any time you need to chill out.

3. Keep your diffuser blend in a cool, dark place between uses.

Tip: No lemon? Try using grapefruit in its place.

HARMONIZING ROLL-ON

TOPICAL, MAY CAUSE PHOTOSENSITIVITY, SAFE FOR CHILDREN AGES 12+

When you're at your wits' end and need to destress—STAT—this roll-on comes to the rescue. The scent is both citrusy and lightly floral, with just a hint of woody frankincense to round things out. MAKES ABOUT 1 TABLESPOON

6 drops frankincense essential oil

12 drops grapefruit essential oil

6 drops lavender essential oil

12 drops Roman chamomile essential oil

1 tablespoon fractionated coconut oil

1. In a roller bottle, combine the frankincense, grapefruit, lavender, and Roman chamomile essential oils with the fractionated coconut oil. Cap the bottle and shake well to combine.

2. Swipe the roller across your wrists and use your fingertips to rub the blend into your hands, inhaling deeply. Take a few minutes to relax, if possible. Repeat as needed.

3. Keep the roll-on in a cool, dark place between applications.

Tip: Try patchouli in place of frankincense, or enjoy the lighter combination of Roman chamomile, grapefruit, and lavender.

Water Retention

Imbalances, damaged capillaries, and a high-salt diet are just a few things that can lead to fluid retention. Aromatherapy can help, especially when you use diuretic oils such as rosemary, lemon, geranium, or grapefruit, and anti-inflammatory oils like lavender, tea tree, or lemongrass. Check with your doctor if you're retaining fluid frequently, as edema can be a symptom of an underlying health condition.

Helpful Essential Oils: geranium, grapefruit, lavender, lemon, lemongrass, patchouli, rosemary, tea tree

SOOTHING SYNERGY BATH

TOPICAL, SAFE FOR CHILDREN AGES 6+

MUST HAVE Geranium, lavender, and rosemary essential oils mingle to create a lovely scent, while helping swollen tissues return to normal. The Epsom salt helps restore balance, too.

MAKES 1 TREATMENT

2 cups Epsom salt

2 drops geranium essential oil

4 drops lavender essential oil

2 drops rosemary essential oil

1. Fill your bathtub with hot water, simultaneously adding the Epsom salt.

2. Add the geranium, lavender, and rosemary essential oils to the bathwater just before you get in. Breathe deeply and relax for at least 15 minutes.

3. Follow up with a Synergistic Tummy Rub (page 106) massage, if needed.

   Tip: Rosemary is a strong stimulant. If you're planning to enjoy this bath at bedtime, omit it or replace it with patchouli essential oil.

REFRESHING CITRUS MASSAGE

TOPICAL, MAY CAUSE PHOTOSENSITIVITY, SAFE FOR AGES 12+

Lemon and grapefruit essential oils are strong diuretics, and using them in a massage blend can help flush excess fluid and relieve swelling. Lemon's analgesic properties make it useful for soothing the discomfort that often accompanies tightly stretched skin.

MAKES ABOUT 2 TABLESPOONS

12 drops grapefruit essential oil

12 drops lemon essential oil

2 tablespoons jojoba oil

1. In a bottle with a tight-fitting cap, combine the grapefruit and lemon essential oils. Let them rest for about 1 hour.

2. Add the jojoba oil, cap the bottle, and shake or swirl to blend completely.

3. With your fingers, apply about ½ teaspoon of the blend to the affected area, using a little more or less as needed. Using gentle strokes, massage in the direction of the heart. If possible, relax with the affected area elevated. Repeat as needed throughout the day.

4. Keep the massage oil in a cool, dark place between uses.

    Tip: If you're missing one of the essential oils for this blend, just double up on the one you do have. You can also create your own blend using any of the recommended essential oils.

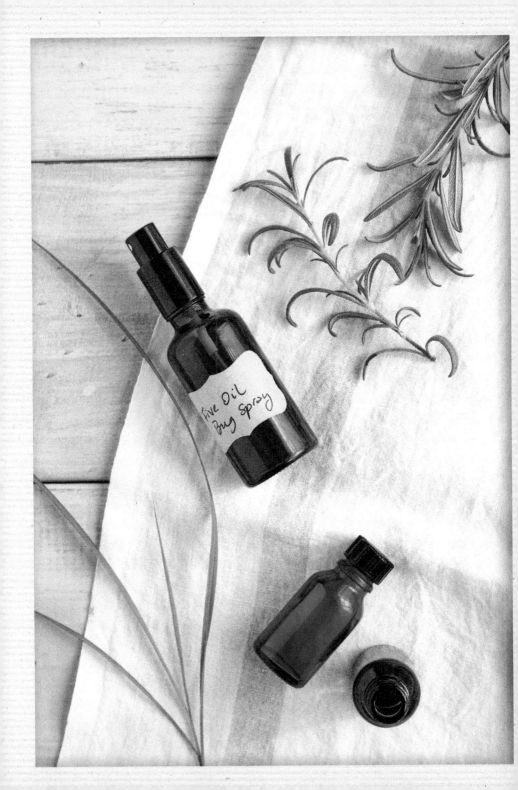

Applications for the Home and Outdoors

S tore shelves are stocked with products designed to deliver cleanliness, freshen air, and more. While the number of natural, ecofriendly solutions is increasing, many products contain dangerous chemicals.

Instead of shelling out for products that have the potential to do more harm than good, why not make a few of your own? This chapter has easy recipes for everything from all-purpose cleaners to DIY laundry detergent that works just as well as the expensive stuff from the store. Insect repellent and pest solutions are found here, too. With simple ingredients and your favorite essential oils, you'll soon be enjoying a clean, chemical-free home.

Air Freshening

Smells from cooking, pets, and everyday life can add up to not-so-fresh indoor air. Instead of reaching for toxic commercial solutions, whip up an aromatherapy blend that removes bacteria from the air, while leaving your home smelling fresh and clean. Simple room sprays, potpourri, and diffuser blends are quick and easy to make, and they're ideal for experimenting with your own fragrance blends.

Helpful Helpful Essential Oils: clary sage, clove, eucalyptus, frankincense, geranium, grapefruit, lavender, lemon, lemongrass, patchouli, peppermint, Roman chamomile, rosemary, tea tree, thyme

LAVENDER-PINE POTPOURRI

AROMATIC, SAFE FOR ALL AGES

MUST HAVE Beautifully symmetrical, pine cones are both natural and decorative, making the ideal vehicle for gently diffusing essential oil. MAKES 1 TREATMENT

20 drops lavender essential oil
¼ cup water

6 to 10 pine cones,
cleaned and dried

1. In a spray bottle, combine the lavender essential oil and water.

2. Place the pine cones in a resealable plastic bag and spray them with the entire contents of the bottle. Seal the bag and leave it closed for at least 24 hours.

3. Place the pine cones in a decorative bowl or basket. Refresh the scent as often as you like by repeating steps 1 and 2.

Tip: You can use this method with a variety of dried natural materials. Flowers, leaves, and cedarwood chips are good choices.

AROMATIC, SAFE FOR ALL AGES

MUST
HAVE

Epsom salt isn't just good for bathing; combined with baking soda and essential oils, it can help keep your home smelling fresh. This easy air freshener is perfect for the bathroom or any area where stinky odors accumulate. MAKES 1 TREATMENT

7 drops clove essential oil	¼ cup Epsom salt
15 drops eucalyptus essential oil	¼ cup baking soda
20 drops lemon essential oil	

1. In a sugar shaker with a perforated lid, combine the clove, eucalyptus, and lemon essential oils with the Epsom salt and baking soda.

2. Set the air freshener in an inconspicuous spot and position the lid so the fragrance is released.

3. Close the lid as needed.

   Tip: When the scent fades, there's no need to make a whole new batch. Simply refresh the salt and baking soda blend with more essential oil.

Ants

Ants are some of nature's hardest-working insects, and they hold an important place in the ecosystem. You've got to draw the line somewhere though; you don't want ants invading your kitchen or garage. Instead of reaching for toxic insecticides, try these natural options instead. Note: You'll need to call in an exterminator if ants are nesting in your walls; natural remedies don't work for a full-scale invasion.

Helpful Essential Oils: clove, eucalyptus, geranium, grapefruit, lemon, lemongrass, peppermint, tea tree

PEPPERMINT ANT BARRIER

AROMATIC, SAFE FOR ALL AGES

MUST HAVE Ants can't stand the smell of peppermint, and they dislike crossing sticky barriers. This remedy uses simple dish soap and peppermint essential oil; with repeated use, ants will look for easier ways to find resources. MAKES ABOUT ½ CUP

40 drops peppermint essential oil

½ cup plain, mildly scented dish soap (Dawn or a similar brand is ideal)

1. In a plastic squeeze bottle, combine the peppermint essential oil and dish soap. Cap the bottle and shake well to blend.

2. Watch the ants to see where they're coming from. Areas such as baseboards, doorways, countertop backsplashes, and window-sills are common entry points.

3. Apply a long line of peppermint-laced dish soap to all areas where you see ants entering and/or leaving your home. Return every hour or so to see if the ants have discovered a new route, and treat that as well.

4. Patience and persistence pay off with this treatment. It might take a few days to find all the ants' trails and treat them. Keep at it; they'll find somewhere else to go.

Tip: Use this treatment in conjunction with Coffee-Clove Ant Barrier for a complete solution.

COFFEE-CLOVE ANT BARRIER

TOPICAL, SAFE FOR ALL AGES

MUST HAVE Clove essential oil has a pungent fragrance that prevents ants from finding and following their pheromone trails. Combined with coffee grounds, which ants also dislike, this remedy creates a barrier to outdoor entry points. MAKES 1 TREATMENT

4 cups dried leftover brewed coffee grounds (see Tip)	20 drops clove essential oil

1. In a large resealable plastic bag, combine the coffee grounds and clove essential oil. Seal the bag and shake well to ensure thorough blending.

2. Look for ant trails outside, around your home's foundation, and around doors and windows. Once you've located the trails, create a one-inch-thick barrier with the clove-coffee grounds.

3. Keep watching for ant activity, and continue applying barriers. If you want to save time, treat the entire perimeter of your home. This calls for more coffee grounds; multiply the recipe as needed and reapply throughout the year to keep ants from invading.

Tip: You can dry the grounds on a baking sheet in a low oven: 200°F for 15 to 20 minutes. If you don't want to save used coffee grounds, use inexpensive ground coffee that hasn't been brewed. Also, you can use any ant-repelling essential oil to create a similar solution.

Dishes

When you add aromatherapy to the mix, the mundane task of doing dishes is a treat for your nose, while the antibacterial oils kill germs without being harsh on your skin. Don't be surprised if you find yourself looking forward to this once-dreaded chore.

Helpful Essential Oils: clove, eucalyptus, grapefruit, lavender, lemon, lemongrass, peppermint, rosemary, tea tree

MINTY LAVENDER-LEMON DISH SOAP

TOPICAL, SAFE FOR ALL AGES

MUST HAVE Lavender, peppermint, and lemon essential oils smell divine together, and this combination increases soap's ability to cut through grease. This blend is a bit less sudsy than commercial types, but works beautifully. MAKES ABOUT 1 CUP

¾ cup liquid castile soap

¼ cup water

20 drops lavender essential oil

20 drops lemon essential oil

6 drops peppermint essential oil

1. In a bottle with a pump top, combine the soap, water, and lavender, lemon, and peppermint essential oils. Cap the bottle and swirl gently to blend.

2. Fill your sink about halfway with comfortably warm water and add about 1 teaspoon of soap. Swish your hand through the sink to create some bubbles, and wash your dishes as usual.

3. Keep the soap in a cool, dark place between uses.

Tip: If you don't like castile soap or you want more bubbles, simply add essential oils to fragrance-free dish soap for a similar experience.

EUCALYPTUS-MINT DISHWASHER SOAP

TOPICAL, SAFE FOR ALL AGES

MUST HAVE Borax is easy to find at most stores that carry cleaning products; it is often located in the laundry aisle. Eucalyptus and peppermint essential oils have a pleasant fragrance, while adding some antibacterial oomph to your dishwasher.
MAKES ABOUT 16 TREATMENTS

1 cup borax

1 cup baking soda

32 drops eucalyptus essential oil

16 drops peppermint essential oil

1. In a large jar with a tight-fitting lid, combine the borax, baking soda, and eucalyptus and peppermint essential oils. Cover the jar and shake to blend well.

2. Use 2 tablespoons of dishwasher soap per load.

3. Keep the soap in a cool, dark place between uses.

   Tip: If you're concerned about spots due to hard water, simply fill your dishwasher's rinse compartment with white vinegar and 1 drop of lemon essential oil.

Fleas

Your home can become infested with fleas even if you don't have indoor pets; these opportunistic insects often hitch rides on human socks, shoes, and pant legs. Natural flea treatments need to be applied frequently; because essential oils don't kill flea eggs, they'll eventually hatch, restarting the life cycle. Exercising patience will help you win this battle without resorting to pesticide use.

Helpful Essential Oils: clove, geranium, lavender, lemongrass, peppermint

LAVENDER-LEMONGRASS FLOOR POWDER

TOPICAL, SAFE FOR ALL AGES

MUST HAVE   Borax, lavender, and lemongrass make short work of adult fleas and larvae. This remedy can be messy, but it's safe for all types of flooring. MAKES ABOUT 2 CUPS

2 cups borax   20 drops lemongrass essential oil
20 drops lavender essential oil

1. In a large jar, combine the borax and lavender and lemongrass essential oils. Cover the jar and shake to mix well.

2. Sprinkle the powder all over your floors, getting it into any cracks and paying particular attention to areas around entryways and baseboards. Leave the treatment in place for 24 hours, and then sweep and vacuum. Repeat once or twice weekly for at least 3 weeks, and again anytime you notice flea activity.

3. Keep the powder in a cool, dark place between uses.

   Tip: You can easily double or triple this recipe if you need to.

LAVENDER-MINT FLEA COLLAR FOR DOGS

AROMATIC, SAFE FOR PUPPIES 8+ WEEKS

MUST HAVE Traditional dog flea collars rely on toxic pesticides. If you're looking for a safer way to repel fleas, try this collar. Note that this is best for pets who spend most of their time indoors, and works best in combination with a comprehensive flea prevention program. Use this flea collar only with dogs, because this blend of essential oils is not safe for cats. MAKES 1 TREATMENT

10 drops lavender essential oil   2 tablespoons sunflower oil
5 drops peppermint essential oil   1 nylon dog collar

1. In a resealable plastic bag, combine the lavender and peppermint essential oils and the sunflower oil.

2. Place the dog collar into the bag. Seal the bag and from the outside, move the collar around so it is coated with oil. Leave the collar in the bag for 24 hours.

3. Put the collar on your dog, preferably after a bath.

   Tip: For a quicker option, apply 4 or 5 drops of lavender essential oil to your dog's collar; the scent can be refreshed at any time.

Floor Care: Rugs and Carpets

Carpeted surfaces feel wonderful on bare feet, plus they provide a bit of soundproofing and insulation. It's easy to keep them fresh and clean with simple aromatherapy products that cost very little to make.

Helpful Essential Oils: clary sage, clove, eucalyptus, frankincense, geranium, grapefruit, lavender, lemon, lemongrass, patchouli, peppermint, Roman chamomile, rosemary, tea tree, thyme

REFRESHING VACUUM POWDER

AROMATIC, SAFE FOR ALL AGES

Tired of paying for chemically scented carpet deodorizers? This simple solution is easy on your budget, particularly when you buy baking soda in bulk. The lavender, grapefruit, lemon, and peppermint essential oils give your home a fresh scent, plus they keep your vacuum cleaner from smelling funky. MAKES ABOUT 2 CUPS

2 cups baking soda
15 drops grapefruit essential oil
15 drops lavender essential oil

10 drops lemon essential oil
5 drops peppermint essential oil

1. In a mixing bowl, combine the baking soda and grapefruit, lavender, lemon, and peppermint essential oils. Use a whisk or fork to blend thoroughly. Transfer the powder to a sugar shaker or jar.

2. Before vacuuming, apply a light dusting of powder over your carpets. Leave the powder in place for at least 5 minutes, and vacuum as usual.

3. Keep the powder in a cool, dark place between uses.

   Tip: This powder can be used for absorbing nonstaining spills on carpets. With paper towels, soak up as much of the spill as you can. Apply a thick coat of powder. Use a stiff brush to scrub it in, and allow the area to dry. Vacuum up the residue.

LEMON STAIN REMOVER

AROMATIC, SAFE FOR ALL AGES

MUST HAVE Instead of reaching for pricey carpet shampoos, try an all-natural solution that leaves a fresh scent behind, while erasing stains. The lemon essential oil, vinegar, and baking soda create plenty of bubbles that lift grime right out of carpet fibers. Note: Use this within about 10 minutes of making it for best results.

MAKES 1 TREATMENT

5 drops lemon essential oil

1 teaspoon dish soap

1 tablespoon white vinegar

1 cup warm water

1½ teaspoons baking soda

1. In a bottle with a spray top, combine the lemon essential oil, dish soap, and vinegar.

2. Add the water and swirl to mix the ingredients.

3. Add the baking soda and cap the bottle quickly. The bubbles may overflow, so do this step over the kitchen sink.

4. Soak the stain with the spray. Use paper towels to blot the area, working from the outer edge to the center of the stain. Repeat.

5. Scrub with a soft brush, working from the outside of the stain to its center. Keep reapplying stain remover and blotting.

6. Allow the area to dry, and vacuum up any residual baking powder.

   Tip: This spray works well on a variety of surfaces, including upholstery and drapes. Test it in an inconspicuous spot before use, just to be sure it will not cause a color change.

Floor Care: Laminate, Linoleum, and Tile

Check out the cleaning aisle in any store and you'll find many options for keeping hard surfaces clean. These work well, but can contain unwanted chemicals, and most are pretty expensive. By putting essential oils to work, these simple options are quick and easy to make, and they're a pleasure to use.

Helpful Essential Oils: clary sage, clove, eucalyptus, frankincense, geranium, grapefruit, lavender, lemon, lemongrass, patchouli, peppermint, Roman chamomile, rosemary, tea tree, thyme

REUSABLE FLOOR SWEEPER WIPES

TOPICAL, SAFE FOR ALL AGES

MUST HAVE Rectangular floor mops with disposable wipes have changed the way many of us clean our floors. Try these wipes the next time you run out of disposables. You may like them better!

MAKES 6 REUSABLE WIPES

6 drops lemon essential oil
6 drops eucalyptus essential oil
¼ cup rubbing alcohol
¼ cup water

¼ cup white vinegar
1 teaspoon dish soap
6 microfiber cleaning cloths,
cut to fit your sweeper

1. In a rectangular storage container with a resealable lid, combine the lemon and eucalyptus essential oils, rubbing alcohol, water, vinegar, and dish soap. Swirl the container gently to blend.

2. Fold the cloths to fit inside the container, and stack them in the cleaning solution. Seal the lid and swish to ensure all cloths are saturated.

3. Attach a cloth to your rectangular mop and clean your floor as usual. Launder the cloths when finished.

4. Keep the wipes in a cool, dark place between uses.

Tip: You can mix up a batch of this floor cleaner and keep it in a spray bottle. Apply it anytime you'd like to spot clean between regular moppings.

AROMATIC, SAFE FOR ALL AGES

MUST HAVE Keep floors looking their best with this polish. It removes residue and brings out shine, leaving a fresh lemon scent behind. MAKES ABOUT 1 CUP

¾ cup plus 1 tablespoon water

1 tablespoon white vinegar

½ teaspoon rubbing alcohol

20 drops lemon essential oil

1. In a microwavable bowl, heat the water nearly to boiling.

2. Add the vinegar and rubbing alcohol. Let the mixture cool completely.

3. Add the lemon essential oil. Use a funnel to transfer the polish to a bottle fitted with a spray top.

4. After sweeping, lightly mist your floors with the polish. Use a soft cloth or a dry mop to go over the polish. Work in sections so you don't slip or leave footprints behind. Repeat as needed.

5. Keep the polish in a cool, dark place between uses.

Tip: This blend is great for spot cleaning a variety of hard surfaces, plus it's nice for bath and shower freshening.

Floor Care: Bamboo, Plank, and Hardwood

Natural wood floors call for special care; you don't want anything harsh that might ruin the finish, nor do you want overly waxy cleaners that leave residue behind. These simple solutions cost very little to make, and they leave your natural wood floors looking and smelling fantastic.

Helpful Essential Oils: clary sage, clove, eucalyptus, frankincense, geranium, grapefruit, lavender, lemon, lemongrass, patchouli, peppermint, Roman chamomile, rosemary, tea tree, thyme

LEMON-MINT FLOOR CLEANER

TOPICAL, SAFE FOR ALL AGES

MUST HAVE Plain dish soap, rubbing alcohol, and vinegar combine with refreshing lemon and peppermint essential oils to leave your floors clean and streak-free, while imparting an invigorating scent.

MAKES ABOUT 1¼ CUPS

12 drops lemon essential oil	1 tablespoon rubbing alcohol
3 drops peppermint essential oil	¼ cup white vinegar
1 teaspoon dish soap	1 cup warm water

1. In a bottle with a spray top, combine the lemon and peppermint essential oils, dish soap, rubbing alcohol, vinegar, and warm water. Cap the bottle and swirl gently to blend.

2. After sweeping, lightly mist your floors with the cleaner. Use a barely damp mop to scrub. Work in sections so you don't slip or leave footprints behind, and rinse your mop as it picks up grime. Repeat as needed.

3. Keep the cleaner in a cool, dark place between uses.

   Tip: If you have a big mopping job, make a double or triple batch of this cleaner right in the mop bucket. Rinse your mop in fresh water and wring it out between dips in the cleanser.

CITRUS FLOOR POLISH

AROMATIC, SAFE FOR ALL AGES

Olive oil and vinegar combine with lemon and grapefruit essential oils to leave natural wood floors clean, shiny, and streak-free. This is a bit labor-intensive but you'll enjoy the results, and get in some citrus aromatherapy while you work. MAKES ABOUT 2 CUPS

10 drops grapefruit essential oil
10 drops lemon essential oil
2 tablespoons olive oil

3 tablespoons white vinegar
1¾ cups hot water

1. In a bucket or bowl, combine the grapefruit and lemon essential oils, olive oil, vinegar, and hot water.

2. With a mop or a soft cloth, apply a very light layer of polish to the floor. You may want to work in sections to prevent tracks.

3. When the floor dries, go over it with a dry dust mop or a dry polishing cloth and remove any excess oil. The more you rub, the better your results will be.

4. Keep any unused polish in a cool, dry place between uses.

   Tip: Around the holidays, add some clove to this blend for a classic, spicy fragrance.

Furniture Care

Wood, metal, and synthetic furnishings look best when they're treated to an occasional polishing. Different materials call for different solutions: Here are two to try next time you're in the mood to give nonupholstered items some TLC.

Helpful Essential Oils: clary sage, clove, eucalyptus, frankincense, geranium, grapefruit, lavender, lemon, lemongrass, patchouli, peppermint, Roman chamomile, rosemary, tea tree, thyme

LAVENDER-LEMON WOOD POLISH

TOPICAL, SAFE FOR ALL AGES

MUST
HAVE
Lavender and lemon essential oils create a wonderful fragrance, while gently cleansing. Avocado oil provides rich, penetrating moisture, and vinegar ensures a streak-free shine. MAKES ABOUT 1 CUP

12 drops lavender essential oil	¼ cup white vinegar
12 drops lemon essential oil	¾ cup avocado oil

1. In a bottle with a tight-fitting top, combine the lavender and lemon essential oils, vinegar, and avocado oil. Cap the bottle and shake well to blend. Shake again before each use.

2. To a soft cloth, apply about ¼ teaspoon of the polish, using a little more or less as needed.

3. Apply the polish to the furniture, working from top to bottom. When you're finished, use another cloth to remove excess and buff to a shine. Repeat every week or two for clean, shiny furniture.

4. Keep the polish in a cool, dry place between uses.

   Tip: No avocado oil? Use olive oil in its place.

GRAPEFRUIT FURNITURE SPRAY

TOPICAL, SAFE FOR ALL AGES

Grapefruit essential oil cuts through grime and leaves a pleasant scent behind. Use this simple cleaning spray to keep metal, plastic, and synthetic leather looking its best. MAKES ABOUT 1 CUP

12 drops grapefruit essential oil	⅓ cup water
1 tablespoon rubbing alcohol	½ cup white vinegar

1. In a bottle fitted with a spray top, combine the grapefruit essential oil, rubbing alcohol, water, and vinegar. Cap the bottle and shake well to blend. Shake again before each use.

2. Apply a light mist of the furniture spray to the item and wipe it down with a soft cloth or paper towel. For spot cleaning, apply a spritz of spray to the cloth or paper towel and use it as needed. Repeat as often as you'd like.

3. Keep the cleaner in a cool, dark, dry place between uses.

   Tip: No grapefruit? Try lemon, eucalyptus, or tea tree essential oil instead.

Garden Diseases

Just like people, plants are susceptible to a variety of diseases. Essential oils come to the rescue, killing fungal infections, stopping mildew, and more. A little goes a long way with plants, particularly when they're young.

Helpful Essential Oils: eucalyptus, lavender, lemon, lemongrass, patchouli, peppermint, tea tree

POWDERY MILDEW SPRAY

TOPICAL, SAFE FOR ALL AGES

Powdery mildew attacks a variety of ornamental plants, and it can often be found in vegetable gardens; I remember one year having all my squash plants covered in the silvery-gray powder. Lemon, patchouli, and tea tree essential oils work well in most cases. MAKES ABOUT 4 CUPS

4 cups water

6 drops lemon essential oil

6 drops patchouli essential oil

6 drops tea tree essential oil

1. In a large spray bottle, combine the water and lemon, patchouli, and tea tree essential oils. Cap the bottle and shake well to blend.

2. Spray all affected areas. Repeat the following day after watering, if necessary.

3. Keep your spray in a cool, dark place between uses.

Tip: Apply the treatment in the evening or on a cloudy day when plants won't be sunburned.

TEA TREE PLANT SPRAY

TOPICAL, SAFE FOR CHILDREN AGES 6+

MUST HAVE If garden plants are ailing and you're not sure of the cause, try treating them with this versatile antifungal spray. It works on a variety of common diseases, early blight on tomato plants, and leather rot on strawberries. You can also apply this as a preventive and use it to clean garden tools after working on diseased plants. MAKES ABOUT 1 CUP

1 tablespoon tea tree essential oil   1 cup distilled water

1. In a spray bottle, combine the tea tree essential oil and distilled water. Cap the bottle and shake well to blend. Shake again before each use.

2. With a sharp pair of garden shears, clip off damaged plant parts. Discard them away from your garden.

3. At dusk or on a cloudy day, apply a light mist of the spray, using just enough to cover the entire plant. If large leaves are present, coat both sides. Repeat every 7 to 12 days to prevent disease.

4. Keep the spray in a cool, dark place between uses.

Tip: Keep your garden weed-free, and do not overwater. Both can increase the likelihood of disease.

Garden Pests

All creatures have important roles to play, but that doesn't mean you have to welcome pests into your garden. Essential oils can protect your harvest and keep your plants healthy by repelling slugs, bugs, and snails that cause harm.

Helpful Essential Oils: clove, geranium, grapefruit, lavender, lemon, lemongrass, patchouli, peppermint, thyme

BUG-BANISHING SYNERGISTIC SPRAY

TOPICAL, SAFE FOR ALL AGES

The d-limonene in citrus essential oils is a potent insecticide, thanks to its ability to dissolve the protective coating that covers insects' exoskeletons. Natural castile soap helps it stick. This spray is effective on a wide range of garden pests, but be careful—it will kill beneficial insects if you accidentally spray them. Use for aphids, ants, whiteflies, squash bugs, and other pests. MAKES ABOUT 1 CUP

1 teaspoon grapefruit essential oil	30 drops peppermint essential oil
60 drops lemon essential oil	1 tablespoon castile soap
	¾ cup water

1. In a spray bottle with a stream setting, combine the grapefruit, lemon, and peppermint essential oils with the soap and water. Cap the bottle and shake to blend well. Shake again before each application.

2. Spray insects directly, preferably after they have landed. Large insects often need 2 or 3 coats of spray, and will often continue moving for a few minutes before dying. Repeat as needed.

3. Keep the spray in a cool, dark place between uses.

   Tip: Trying to win the war against squash bugs? Look under leaves and kill tiny hatchlings. Check for pests daily.

PATCHOULI SLUG BARRIER

TOPICAL, SAFE FOR ALL AGES

If you're finding little holes in your lettuce leaves, it's likely slugs and snails are treating your garden as a salad bar. This simple treatment calls for coffee and patchouli essential oil. As a bonus, the coffee nourishes garden soil and the patchouli helps keep other pests away from your plants. MAKES 1 TREATMENT

1 large (about 30.5-ounce) can regular ground coffee, any brand

20 drops patchouli essential oil

1. Open the coffee can and add the patchouli essential oil to the grounds. Use a fork or similar utensil to blend well.

2. Lay a 1-inch coffee barrier around slug- and snail-sensitive plants. You can treat individual plants or surround entire rows or sections. Reapply once or twice a week.

3. Keep the covered can in a cool place between uses.

Tip: Don't use decaffeinated coffee for this treatment. Part of the reason this treatment works so well is that slugs and snails have a natural aversion to caffeine.

Healthy Houseplants

Houseplants add beauty to your home, while helping keep indoor air clean, but they're susceptible to fungal infections, or can gather dust on their leaves. These treatments are quick, easy, and help your houseplants live up to their natural potential.

Helpful Essential Oils: eucalyptus, lavender, lemon, lemongrass, patchouli, peppermint, tea tree

IMMUNITY WATERING TREATMENT

TOPICAL, SAFE FOR ALL AGES

MUST HAVE Added to the soil, lavender essential oil prevents fungal growth and helps plants stay healthy. A little goes a long way. If you accidentally add extra drops, increase the amount of water in your blend to prevent overexposure. MAKES 1 GALLON

4 drops lavender essential oil   1 gallon water

1. In a watering can, combine the lavender essential oil and water.

2. Water your houseplants as usual. Repeat the treatment every third or fourth watering to keep fungus from developing.

Tip: If a plant develops a fungal infection, mix up a spray with 8 drops lavender essential oil to 1 gallon water, and mist it onto the plant once daily. If the affected plant is kept in close proximity to other houseplants, you may want to mist them as a preventive measure.

LEMONGRASS LEAF POLISH

AROMATIC, SAFE FOR ALL AGES

MUST HAVE You may have heard that olive oil or mayonnaise brings out the shine on plant leaves, but these treatments can do more harm than good, attracting pests and leaving residue behind. This spray supports healthy plants naturally, plus removes tiny pests such as spider mites. MAKES ABOUT ½ CUP

2 drops lemongrass essential oil   ¼ cup plus 2 tablespoons
¼ teaspoon castile soap   distilled water
1 tablespoon white vinegar

1. In a bottle fitted with a spray top, combine the lemongrass essential oil, soap, vinegar, and water. Cap the bottle and shake to blend completely.

2. Apply a light mist to your houseplant and use a soft cloth or a clean cosmetics brush to remove any debris or dust from the leaves. Wipe the leaves' undersides and stems, if needed, and mist the whole plant with distilled water. Repeat every week or two.

3. Keep the spray in a cool, dark place between uses.

   Tip: No lemongrass? Use any houseplant-appropriate essential oil; lemon and grapefruit are excellent options.

Insect Repellent

Read the ingredients list on a bug spray container and you might be shocked by the number of unpronounceable chemicals. While many companies produce all-natural insect repellents, it's just as easy to make your own.

Helpful Essential Oils: clary sage, clove, eucalyptus, geranium, lavender, lemongrass, patchouli, peppermint, rosemary, tea tree

FIVE-OIL BUG SPRAY

TOPICAL, SAFE FOR CHILDREN AGES 2+

MUST HAVE Five of the most powerful insect-repelling essential oils come together in this spray, which smells much nicer than the commercial stuff, while offering effective protection from a variety of biting bugs. The aloe and glycerin are optional, but they help the repellent stay on your skin longer, and offer natural moisture.

MAKES ABOUT 1 CUP

30 drops eucalyptus essential oil	¼ cup water
30 drops geranium essential oil	1 tablespoon rubbing alcohol
20 drops lavender essential oil	1 tablespoon aloe vera gel
30 drops lemongrass essential oil	(optional)
15 drops rosemary essential oil	1 teaspoon vegetable glycerin
½ cup alcohol-free witch hazel	(optional)

1. In a bottle fitted with a spray top, combine the eucalyptus, gera-nium, lavender, lemongrass, and rosemary essential oils.

2. Add the witch hazel, water, rubbing alcohol, and aloe vera gel and glycerin (if using). Cap the bottle and shake well to combine. Shake again before each use.

3. Spritz a light layer onto areas of exposed skin, and reapply as needed.

4. Keep the insect repellent in a cool, dark place between uses.

Tip: Make this spray your own and create a scent that appeals to you with any combination of insect-repelling essential oils. Or whip up a quick version with water and oils alone. The other ingredients are nice to have, but aren't necessary repel-ling bugs.

BUGS BE GONE LOTION

TOPICAL, SAFE FOR CHILDREN AGES 2+

Treat your skin to some much-needed moisture, while experienc-ing an insect repellent that smells more like an elegant perfume than a traditional bug spray. Thanks to your favorite fragrance-free lotion, this recipe is easy. MAKES ABOUT 1 CUP

60 drops frankincense essential oil

20 drops lemongrass essential oil

40 drops patchouli essential oil

1 cup fragrance-free lotion

1. In a small glass bottle with a tight-fitting lid, combine the frank-incense, lemongrass, and patchouli essential oils. Let them rest overnight.

2. In a small bowl, combine the lotion and essential oil blend. Use a utensil, such as a fork or whisk, to blend thoroughly. Transfer the lotion to a jar with a tight-fitting lid.

3. With your fingertips, apply a dime-sized amount to each area of exposed skin, using a little more or less as needed. Reapply when the fragrance fades or if bugs start to bother you.

4. Keep the lotion in a cool, dark place between uses.

Tip: If you don't have lemongrass, try geranium or lavender essential oil.

Kitchen and Bath Countertops

Countertops are hard-working surfaces, and they tend to get grimy fast. Essential oils cut through grease and dirt, and kill bacteria naturally.

Helpful Essential Oils: clove, eucalyptus, lavender, lemon, lemongrass, patchouli, peppermint, rosemary, tea tree

LEMON-EUCALYPTUS CLEANSER

TOPICAL, SAFE FOR ALL AGES

MUST HAVE Fresh-smelling eucalyptus combines with lemon essential oil, creating an uplifting aroma, while banishing germs in the kitchen and bath. This cleanser contains vinegar, so it isn't safe for stone countertops. MAKES ABOUT 1 CUP

8 drops eucalyptus essential oil	½ cup white vinegar
20 drops lemon essential oil	½ cup water
2 drops dish soap	

1. In a bottle fitted with a spray top, combine the eucalyptus and lemon essential oils, dish soap, vinegar, and water. Cap the bottle and shake to blend. Shake again before each use.

2. Mist a light coating of spray onto countertops and wipe clean with a paper towel or cloth. Repeat as needed.

3. Keep the cleanser in a cool, dark place between uses.

Tip: If you have a stubborn, sticky spot, dampen it with this spray and top it with a pinch of baking soda. Wait until the bubbling subsides, and wipe.

GRANITE-SAFE COUNTERTOP CLEANSER

TOPICAL, SAFE FOR ALL AGES

MUST HAVE This mild cleanser is safe for most stone countertops including granite, and it's far less expensive than the commercial versions. Tea tree, lavender, and eucalyptus essential oils offer an appealing fragrance, while sanitizing countertops.

MAKES ABOUT 1 CUP

2 drops eucalyptus essential oil

6 drops lavender essential oil

2 drops tea tree essential oil

2 drops castile soap

2 tablespoons rubbing alcohol

¾ cup plus 1 tablespoon water

1. In a bottle fitted with a spray top, combine the eucalyptus, lavender, and tea tree essential oils, soap, rubbing alcohol and water. Cap the bottle and shake to blend. Shake again before each use.

2. Mist a light coating of spray onto countertops and wipe clean with a paper towel or cloth.

3. Keep your countertop cleanser in a cool, dark place between uses.

Tip: For stubborn, dried on-spots, apply a spritz of cleansing spray and add a pinch of table salt. Gently rub to remove the stain and wipe clean.

Laundry

Eco-friendly laundry solutions are becoming more popular, but can be more expensive than others. If you'd rather keep your cash for something else, give these solutions a try.

Helpful Essential Oils: clary sage, clove, eucalyptus, frankincense, geranium, grapefruit, lavender, lemon, lemongrass, patchouli, peppermint, Roman chamomile, rosemary, tea tree, thyme

LAVENDER-LEMONGRASS LAUNDRY DETERGENT

TOPICAL, SAFE FOR ALL AGES

MUST HAVE This laundry soap smells fantastic, plus the lavender and lemongrass essential oils kill the bacteria that can accumulate in the washing machine. I use a solid soap for this recipe; it, along with the borax and the washing soda can be found in the laundry or cleaning aisle at most big-box stores. MAKES ENOUGH FOR 32 LOADS

20 drops lavender essential oil

20 drops lemongrass essential oil

1 cup borax

1 cup washing soda

2 cups grated vegetable soap

(about 1½ bars)

1. In an airtight tub or large jar, combine the lavender and lemongrass essential oils and borax. Using a fork or similar utensil, stir to combine.

2. Add the washing soda and stir again.

3. Add the grated soap and stir until all ingredients are well combined.

4. If you use cold water for washing, consider running the soap through your food processer, using the regular blade attachment to transform it into a finer powder so it will dissolve easier.

5. Add 2 tablespoons of the laundry detergent to your washing machine's soap compartment and run your load as usual.

6. For extra softness, fill the liquid fabric softener compartment with white vinegar before running the machine.

7. Keep the laundry detergent in a cool, dark, and dry place between uses.

   Tip: If you have a food processer with a grater attachment, use it to speed up the task of prepping the soap.

LAVENDER-MINT DRYER SHEETS

AROMATIC, SAFE FOR ALL AGES

MUST HAVE There are lots of uses for microfiber cloths; in the dryer, they can take the place of toxic dryer sheets by carrying essential oils that impart a light fragrance to clothing. This won't soften your clothes, though, so add vinegar to the wash cycle for added softness without chemicals. MAKES 1 TREATMENT

3 drops lavender essential oil   2 drops peppermint essential oil

1. To a microfiber cloth, add the lavender and peppermint essential oils.

2. Toss the cloth into the dryer with your clothing and dry as usual.

   Tip: Some fragrance will evaporate in the dryer. If you like the blend and want to increase the amount of scent that remains on your laundry, mix up a quick linen spray. Use twice the amount of essential oil and about ½ cup water, and spritz onto dry clothing.

Linens

Treating linens such as sheets, towels, and tablecloths to special care might seem old-fashioned, but the results are worth a few extra minutes of attention. If you're in a pinch for time, try creating linen sprays with your favorite aromatherapy blends. Your whole home will smell more fragrant, and you'll find even more pleasure in the simple act of toweling yourself off or climbing into bed after a long day.

Helpful Essential Oils: clary sage, clove, eucalyptus, frankincense, geranium, grapefruit, lavender, lemon, lemongrass, patchouli, peppermint, Roman chamomile, rosemary, tea tree, thyme

LAVENDER LINEN SPRAY

AROMATIC, SAFE FOR ALL AGES

MUST HAVE Not many people iron clothes these days. Next time you want to enjoy the luxury of freshly ironed clothes or table linens, though, treat yourself to a quick aromatherapy session, while imparting a lovely scent. MAKES ABOUT 1 CUP

30 drops lavender essential oil   1 cup distilled water

1. In a bottle fitted with a spray top, combine the lavender essential oil and distilled water. Cap the bottle and shake well before use. Shake again if you notice the lavender floating to the top during use.

2. Set your iron's temperature to the appropriate level for the fabric you're ironing.

3. Lightly spritz your items and iron them.

4. Keep the linen spray in a cool, dark place between uses.

   Tip: Use distilled water for this recipe; minerals can leave residue behind on fabric and cause discoloration.

LEMON-CLOVE WRINKLE RELEASER

AROMATIC, SAFE FOR ALL AGES

MUST HAVE Why pay a bundle for wrinkle releaser when you can make your own? This fantastic fabric care spray has an appealing, fresh scent that most people enjoy. Don't worry about the vinegar; its odor evaporates quickly. MAKES ABOUT 1 CUP

6 drops clove essential oil

20 drops lemon essential oil

1 teaspoon fragrance-free
(hair) conditioner

1½ teaspoons vinegar

1 cup water

1. In a bottle fitted with a spray top, combine the clove and lemon essential oils, conditioner, vinegar, and water. Cap the bottle and shake to blend. Shake again before each use.

2. Apply a spritz to wrinkled clothing and rub the wrinkled areas with your fingertips. Repeat as needed. Tough wrinkles may require multiple applications.

3. Keep the wrinkle releaser in a cool, dark, dry place between uses.

Tip: You can use any essential oil or blend that appeals to you, and enjoy some psychological benefits while helping your clothes look their best.

Mice and Rats

Rodents don't mean you any harm, but they do carry diseases and can carry pests such as ticks and fleas. Traps are inhumane and poison can harm animals that eat rodents, plus it's another toxin you probably don't want around. Instead, try aromatherapy. Scents that appeal to us are often excellent for repelling mice, rats, and other rodents.

Helpful Essential Oils: grapefruit, lemon, peppermint

PEPPERMINT RODENT BOMBS

AROMATIC, SAFE FOR ALL AGES

MUST HAVE   Peppermint is tough on rodents; they avoid it at all costs. You'll have to stay on top of things when you use this treatment, since the peppermint evaporates quickly. Once rodents figure out they're not welcome, though, they will look for an easier target. MAKES 1 TREATMENT

1 (15-ml) bottle (about 1 tablespoon) peppermint essential oil	1 bag (about 200 to 300) cotton balls

1. Fill an airtight container with a lid, such as a Mason jar, with the cotton balls.

2. Add the entire bottle of peppermint essential oil to the cotton balls. Use a narrow spatula or similar tool to distribute the oil evenly in the container.

3. Close the container and let the cotton balls sit in the jar for 24 hours, to pick up as much scent as possible.

4. Tuck cotton balls into areas where you have noticed rodent activity. Check the balls every few days to be sure they still have a minty smell, and replace as needed.

5. Keep any unused bombs in a cool, dark place between uses.

   Tip: Consider planting peppermint as part of your landscaping. Its odor will repel outdoor mice looking for shelter, and fewer rodents will find their way into your home.

LEMON-MINT RODENT REPELLENT

AROMATIC, SAFE FOR ALL AGES

MUST HAVE Diatomaceous earth is a natural powder sourced from sedimentary rock made up of the shells of prehistoric organisms. Its particles have sharp edges that cut through insect shells and bother rodents, but does not harm humans or pets. Adding essential oils to diatomaceous earth creates an excellent rodent repellent that is easy to pour into holes and hideaways. You can use this indoors and out; look for diatomaceous earth at your local garden shop or online. MAKES ABOUT 2 CUPS

| 10 drops lemon essential oil | ¼ cup water |
| 20 drops peppermint essential oil | 2 cups diatomaceous earth |

1. In a large airtight container, combine the lemon and peppermint essential oils and water.

2. Add the diatomaceous earth, a little at a time, using a sturdy utensil, such as a spatula, to blend.

3. Add more water if needed; the entire batch should be lightly damp when finished. The blend will dry out over time, which is fine; the water is there to ensure the essential oils penetrate the diatomaceous earth.

4. Apply a 1-inch-wide barrier to areas where you've noticed rodent activity, and push the treated diatomaceous earth into any mouse holes or access points you find. Repeat as needed, usually every 5 to 7 days until rodent activity subsides.

5. Store the unused portion in a cool, dark place between uses.

Tip: If it's been a while since you used your rodent repellent and the scent has faded, refresh it by adding more water and essential oil to the container.

Moths and Beetles

Chewing moths and beetles can cause quite a bit of damage. While aromatherapy won't eliminate a full-blown infestation, you can use a variety of essential oils to prevent these bothersome pests from seeking shelter.

Helpful Essential Oils: clove, eucalyptus, geranium, grapefruit, lemon, lemongrass, peppermint, tea tree, thyme

CINNAMON-CLOVE MOTH REPELLENT

AROMATIC, SAFE FOR ALL AGES

MUST HAVE Different essential oils work on different insects, but clove seems to be universally hated. This is a very simple treatment that leaves closets smelling fresh. MAKES 10 STICKS

100 drops clove essential oil   10 cinnamon sticks

1. On a cookie sheet lined with parchment paper, arrange the cinnamon sticks.

2. Add 10 drops of clove essential oil to each cinnamon stick and drop the sticks into a jar with a tight-fitting lid. To be most effective, the scented cinnamon sticks should be used right away.

3. To use, place 1 or 2 cinnamon sticks into a sugar shaker with a perforated lid. Place the shaker in the closet or in other areas that attract moths.

4. Periodically refresh the cinnamon sticks with more clove oil; every 2 to 4 weeks should do the trick.

Tip: Many moths lay their eggs in carpeting, and pantry moths are attracted to open containers of starchy food. For prevention, vacuum at least once each week, and don't leave food packages open.

ALL-PURPOSE BEETLE POWDER

TOPICAL, SAFE FOR ALL AGES

Carpet beetles, cigarette beetles, and drugstore beetles can make their way into the cleanest of homes via packages of food and other dry goods. Other bugs come in via minuscule cracks. This powder calls for grapefruit essential oil and diatomaceous earth, two natural substances that kill insects. MAKES ABOUT 2 CUPS

40 drops grapefruit essential oil	2 cups diatomaceous earth
¼ cup water	(food-grade if treating
	a pantry)

1. In a large airtight container, combine the grapefruit essential oil and water.

2. Add the diatomaceous earth, a little at a time, using a sturdy utensil, such as a spatula, to blend. Add more water if needed; the entire batch should be lightly damp when finished. The blend will dry out over time, which is fine; the water is there to ensure the essential oils penetrate the diatomaceous earth.

3. Sprinkle the blend in areas where you've noticed insect activity. Leave the diatomaceous earth in place for at least 24 hours and then vacuum it up. Reapply as needed.

4. Store the blend in a cool, dark place between uses.

Tip: Leave your diatomaceous earth treatment in place if you're treating cracks and crevices where insects enter and/or hide. It's nontoxic and will keep working for weeks.

Ovens and Microwaves

You don't have to use toxic products to keep appliances clean; instead, treat them to frequent, gentle cleansings using natural solutions. I love knowing I'll never again find myself gagging over the wretched stench of oven cleaner, and I bet you will, too.

Helpful Essential Oils: clary sage, clove, eucalyptus, geranium, grapefruit, lavender, lemon, lemongrass, patchouli, Roman chamomile, rosemary, tea tree, thyme

LEMON-FRESH OVEN CLEANER

TOPICAL, SAFE FOR ALL AGES

MUST HAVE Lemon essential oil and dish soap cut through grease, while baking soda and vinegar penetrate burnt-on goop. Pick a day when you're not planning to use the oven for cooking, because this process can take a while. MAKES 1 TREATMENT

12 drops lemon essential oil	¼ cup white vinegar
2 tablespoons dish soap	1 ¼ cups baking soda

1. In a glass bowl, combine the lemon essential oil, dish soap, vinegar, and baking soda.

2. Add enough hot water to form a thick paste.

3. Remove the oven racks from the oven. (When you're done cleaning the oven, you can also use the cleaner on the racks, if needed.)

4. With a damp cloth, apply the cleaner onto the soiled areas of the oven. Let the cleaner stay in place for at least 8 hours; for heavy soil, leave it on overnight.

5. Use hot water and a sponge to wipe the oven clean. A rough-textured scrubber may prove useful on tough spots.

Tip: After cleaning your oven, consider protecting the bottom with a silicone mat. You'll still want to scrub your oven occasionally to keep it clean, but the mat will catch big spills and make them easy to eliminate.

GRAPEFRUIT MICROWAVE STEAM

TOPICAL, SAFE FOR ALL AGES

If you've ever had a bowl of spaghetti sauce splatter all over the inside of your microwave, you know how tough it can be to clean. Steam and grease-cutting grapefruit essential oil make this dreaded chore simple—whether your mess is large or small. MAKES 1 TREATMENT

2 cups water   6 drops grapefruit essential oil

1. If you've had a big spill, clean up as much as you can.

2. In a large microwave-safe bowl or pie plate, add the water.

3. Microwave on high power to bring the water to a boil.

4. Add the grapefruit essential oil and shut the door. Leave the microwave off and let the water steam inside for at least 5 minutes.

5. Remove the bowl and use a cloth or paper towels to wipe the interior of the microwave. You can use a little bit of the grapefruit solution if you need to go over any spots again.

Tip: Pour the water down the sink with the garbage disposer running. Congratulations! You've just cleaned and freshened two notorious grunge magnets with one simple treatment.

Sinks, Showers, and Toilets

All sorts of debris makes its way down the drains in your home, and germs find safe havens in microscopic cracks and crevices that cover many surfaces. These cleansers are completely nontoxic, yet they do an outstanding job of sanitizing hardworking fixtures.

Helpful Essential Oils: clary sage, clove, eucalyptus, geranium, grapefruit, lavender, lemon, lemongrass, patchouli, Roman chamomile, rosemary, tea tree, thyme

THIEVES-INSPIRED CLEANSING SPRAY

TOPICAL, SAFE FOR ALL AGES

MUST HAVE "Thieves" is a classic herbal blend inspired by tales of robbers who stole from plague victims centuries ago. Its germ-killing power and fresh, appealing scent make it a must-have for a variety of natural cleaning applications. MAKES ABOUT 1 CUP

10 drops clove essential oil	4 drops rosemary essential oil
6 drops eucalyptus essential oil	6 drops tea tree essential oil
10 drops lavender essential oil	¼ cup rubbing alcohol
10 drops lemon essential oil	¾ cup water

1. In a bottle fitted with a spray top, combine the clove, eucalyptus, lavender, lemon, rosemary, and tea tree essential oils, rubbing alcohol, and water. Cap the bottle and shake well to blend. Shake again before each use.

2. Mist the area to be cleaned. Use paper towels or a sanitized cleaning tool, such as a sponge or brush, to clean the area. Repeat for heavier soil. Use as often as you'd like to keep your entire home clean and fresh, naturally.

3. Store your cleanser in a cool, dark place between uses.

   Tip: No rubbing alcohol? Don't fret. It helps kill germs faster, while emulsifying the blend, but it isn't necessary; just replace it with an equal amount of water or witch hazel for similar results.

LEMON-EUCALYPTUS SOFT SCRUB

TOPICAL, SAFE FOR ALL AGES

MUST HAVE Get sinks, showers, and toilets sparkling clean with this all-natural soft scrub made with mildly abrasive baking soda that slowly dissolves instead of eroding surfaces. The lemon and eucalyptus essential oils add germ-fighting power to this blend.

MAKES ABOUT 1 CUP

12 drops eucalyptus essential oil	1 cup baking soda
15 drops lemon essential oil	¼ to ½ cup water
1 tablespoon dish soap	

1. In a jar with a tight-fitting lid, combine the eucalyptus and lemon essential oils, dish soap, and baking soda. Use a thin utensil to stir in enough water to create a consistency that appeals to you.

2. With a clean sponge, brush, or cloth, apply about 1 tablespoon of the scrub to the area to be cleaned; using a little more or less as needed. Scrub thoroughly, and use warm water to rinse. Tough soap scum and similar grime might require two or more applications. Repeat as often as you like.

3. Keep the scrub in a cool, dark place between uses.

   Tip: Got mildew? Apply a thin layer of this scrub and let it sit for about 10 minutes. Scrub with a soft brush and mildew should disappear. Deeply embedded mildew stains may call for a stronger commercial solution, such as bleach.

Upholstery

Upholstered furniture and vehicle interiors call for special care. While it's definitely tempting to reach for commercial solutions, these natural upholstery cleaners usually do the trick. Note that old stains or very large spills might call for professional attention.

Helpful Essential Oils: clary sage, eucalyptus, geranium, lavender, patchouli, Roman chamomile, rosemary, tea tree

EUCALYPTUS UPHOLSTERY SPRAY

TOPICAL, SAFE FOR ALL AGES

MUST HAVE Like commercial cleaning sprays, this contains plenty of rubbing alcohol, a powerful solvent. Vinegar cuts through grease, and eucalyptus essential oil contributes antibacterial action, while leaving a fresh scent behind. MAKES ABOUT 1 CUP

24 drops eucalyptus essential oil   ½ cup white vinegar
½ cup rubbing alcohol

1. In a bottle fitted with a spray top, combine the eucalyptus essential oil, rubbing alcohol, and vinegar. Cap the bottle and shake well to blend. Shake again before each use.

2. Spray the stain and allow the blend to absorb for about 1 minute.

3. Scrub vigorously with a textured towel, working your way from the outer edge of the stain to its center. Re-apply and continue scrubbing until the stain is gone.

4. Keep the upholstery spray in a cool, dark place between uses.

Tip: If there is any dirt or debris on the upholstery, vacuum or brush it off before beginning.

LEMON-GERANIUM LEATHER CLEANER

TOPICAL, SAFE FOR ALL AGES

MUST HAVE Test this first on a hidden area and let it sit for about 15 minutes to be sure the cleaner is right for you. Be careful: Suede and some other leather products get darker with exposure to natural oils. MAKES ABOUT 1 CUP

5 drops geranium essential oil	½ cup olive oil
20 drops lemon essential oil	½ cup white vinegar

1. In a bottle with a tight-fitting lid, combine the geranium and lemon essential oils, olive oil, and vinegar. Cap the bottle and shake well before use, and shake frequently while cleaning leather.

2. Vacuum the item to be cleaned, and wipe it with a damp cloth or paper towel.

3. On a soft cloth or paper towel, apply about ½ teaspoon of leather cleaner. Quickly rub the cleaner onto the item, and use a second clean cloth or paper towel to rub off any excess and buff the leather to a shine. Repeat as often as you like. Frequent conditioning keeps leather soft and supple, so it lasts longer.

4. Keep your leather cleaner in a cool, dark place between uses.

Tip: Tempted to leave the vinegar out of the equation? Don't! It cuts through dirt and helps the oil penetrate.

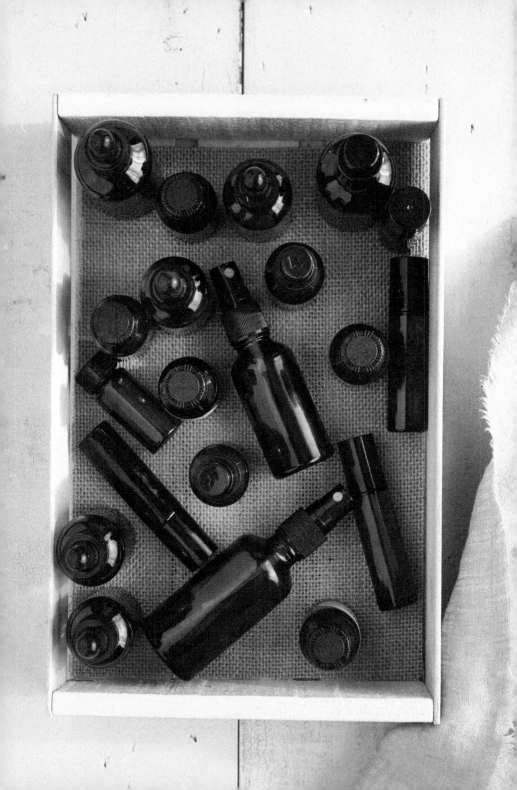

Measurements and Conversions

Since there are a number of differences in tools, utensils, and drop sizes, and variances in judgment from one user to the next, these conversions and measurements should be considered approximations. Some are used in recipes and examples within this book. Others are used in different aromatherapy texts.

1 ml = 20 drops = 0.33 ounce = 0.27 dram

1 teaspoon = 1 dram = 75 drops = ⅛ ounce = 3.7 ml

15 ml = 1 tablespoon = 300 drops = 0.5 ounce = ½ ounce

3 teaspoons = 1 tablespoon

2 tablespoons = 1 ounce

16 tablespoons = 8 ounces = 1 cup

2 cups = 1 pint

4 cups = 1 quart

4 quarts = 1 gallon

Popular Synergy Blends

When mixed together, certain essential oils create synergy blends that offer better results than single oils on their own. Synergy blends are unique chemical compounds you can use for a variety of purposes; some magnify specific essential oil benefits, such as relaxation, pain relief, or skin healing, and others offer pleasing scents for use around the holidays or in home and body care applications.

Most essential oil manufacturers offer their own synergy blends. Some brands carry just a few, while others offer many fantastic combinations. Experiment with creating your own synergy blends, too. Here are ten of the most popular blends to help you get started.

Making and Storing Synergy Blends

The best way to make and store synergy blends is to obtain (or recycle your empty) dark-colored essential oil bottles. Unless you make very large batches, the 15 ml (1 tablespoon) size should suffice.

Mix the blend in the bottle, cap it tightly, and let it rest for at least 24 hours before you use it.

When you're ready to use the blend, add it to your diffuser or use the dilution guide (see page 34) to create safe, effective recipes for a variety of purposes.

Better Digestion

Many essential oils support healthy digestion and alleviate digestive discomfort. This works well whether you have all the oils or not; if you're missing one, try it anyway. Diffuse this blend, or create a soothing abdominal massage using the dilution guide.

- 40 drops lemon essential oil
- 40 drops lemongrass essential oil
- 20 drops patchouli essential oil
- 60 drops peppermint essential oil

Breathe Easy

Stuffy sinuses call for a quick response. Breathing blends typically contain crisply scented essential oils that support respiratory health. This blend is very powerful; start with 2 or 3 drops and add more if you feel you need stronger action. Omit the rosemary essential oil if you plan to use this synergy blend at bedtime. Try diffusing this blend, or add a few drops to your bath or shower for soothing relief.

- 40 drops eucalyptus essential oil
- 40 drops peppermint essential oil
- 20 drops rosemary essential oil
- 40 drops tea tree essential oil

Calm, Cool, and Collected

If you simply want to relax, this easygoing blend will help you! While it's less complex than some of the most popular synergy blends for de-stressing, it promotes relaxation so you can unwind. Try diffusing this blend, or dilute it in your favorite carrier oil for topical use.

- 50 drops clary sage essential oil
- 50 drops lavender essential oil
- 20 drops patchouli essential oil
- 50 drops Roman chamomile essential oil

Detox

Most essential oils offer detoxifying benefits, and there are dozens of popular synergy blends to choose from. This one makes good use of some of the most common, least expensive oils. Try diffusing this blend, or dilute it in carrier oil for a soothing leg massage.

- 50 drops grapefruit essential oil
- 50 drops lemon essential oil
- 30 drops peppermint essential oil
- 20 drops rosemary essential oil

Inner Peace

Harmonizing synergy blends are ideal for meditating, relaxing, or creating a carefree atmosphere in your home. This blend is far simpler than the complex ones offered for sale by top distributors, and it's ideal for diffusing when you're relaxing or meditating.

- 20 drops clary sage essential oil
- 50 drops frankincense essential oil
- 10 drops geranium essential oil
- 20 drops lavender essential oil
- 10 drops lemon essential oil
- 20 drops Roman chamomile essential oil

Joyful

Create a happy, joyous atmosphere in your home by diffusing a synergistic blend that contains plenty of citrus and just a little spice. Some popular blends also incorporate a touch of floral fragrance, which adds even more luxury.

- 10 drops clove essential oil
- 60 drops grapefruit essential oil
- 15 drops lavender essential oil
- 60 drops lemon essential oil

Mental Clarity

Whether you're working, studying, or engaging in a demanding task, a mental clarity blend can help. Most of these blends contain rosemary, citrus, and other energizing essential oils. Try diffusing this blend, or add a few drops to your favorite piece of aromatherapy jewelry.

- 20 drops eucalyptus essential oil
- 10 drops geranium essential oil
- 40 drops grapefruit oil
- 40 drops lemon essential oil
- 40 drops rosemary essential oil

Peaceful Sleep

When you're ready to end the day, synergy blends designed to promote peaceful sleep can help you unwind and drift off. Diffuse them, apply them to your pillowcase, or use them in bedtime bath and body products.

- 40 drops clary sage essential oil
- 5 drops geranium essential oil
- 50 drops lavender essential oil
- 10 drops lemon essential oil
- 2 drops peppermint essential oil

Quick Pain Relief

Pain relief blends typically include hot, deeply penetrating oils, and many brands add calming essential oils to help provide relief from mental. Try diluting this blend with a carrier oil and using it to massage sore joints or painful muscles.

- 20 drops clove essential oil
- 20 drops eucalyptus essential oil
- 40 drops lavender essential oil
- 40 drops peppermint essential oil
- 40 drops Roman chamomile essential oil
- 40 drops thyme essential oil

Thieves

There are many versions of the popular thieves, or four thieves, blend. This one is simple to make, and it is excellent for a variety of cleaning and freshening applications.

- 40 drops clove essential oil
- 24 drops eucalyptus essential oil
- 40 drops lavender essential oil
- 40 drops lemon essential oil
- 24 drops rosemary essential oil
- 16 drops tea tree essential oil

Resources

When you begin to research the subject of aromatherapy, you'll discover there are countless sources of useful information. This is a short list that includes some of my favorite books, websites, and organizations, each with plenty of wisdom to impart. It was a challenge to create such a short list; if not limited by space, this little directory would be much longer.

Websites

Base Formula Aromatherapy: baseformula-us.com
Base Formula offers a wide range of products including essential oils, hydrosols, and more. The site also features an informative blog, videos, and more.

Bulk Apothecary: bulkapothecary.com
Packaging, labels, and excellent ingredients are just some of the things you'll find at Bulk Apothecary. Beautiful herbs to add to your remedies, candle- and soap-making supplies, and many other exciting treasures are found here.

Dreaming Earth Botanicals: dreamingearth.com
Dreaming Earth offers unique diffusers, lovely storage boxes to protect your essential oils, and plenty of ingredients to go into your recipes. The company offers lots of inspiration via its blog, recipes, and FAQ section.

Mountain Rose Herbs: mountainroseherbs.com
While the company's name might lead you to believe that only herbs are on the menu, Mountain Rose Herbs offers an extensive selection of supplies for making your own remedies. Recipes, an excellent blog, and frequent sales make this a must-visit.

Rocky Mountain Oils: rockymountainoils.com
Affectionately known as RMO, Rocky Mountain Oils offers an impressive selection of essential oils, blends, and accessories.

Starwest Botanicals: starwest-botanicals.com
You'll find plenty of accessories, natural body care products, herbal extracts, and essential oils at Starwest Botanicals. This company has been in business since 1975, and offers thousands of products.

Books

Lawless, Julia. *The Illustrated Encyclopedia of Essential Oils: The Complete Guide to the Use of Oils in Aromatherapy and Herbalism.* New York City: HarperCollins, 1995.
If you want to dig deep into the practice of aromatherapy, consider this book. It profiles more than 160 essential oils in depth, and will expand your knowledge greatly.

Tisserand, Robert B. *The Art of Aromatherapy: The Healing and Beautifying Properties of the Essential Oils of Flowers and Herbs.* New York City: Simon & Schuster (Healing Arts Press), 1978.
One of the most definitive guides to the practice of aromatherapy, this book holds a place of honor on my shelf and those of many others. The book was published in 1978, but the information it contains remains relevant even decades later.

Tisserand, Robert, and Rodney Young. *Essential Oil Safety: A Guide for Health Care Professionals.* 2nd ed. Edinburgh: Churchill Livingstone, 2013.

Robert Tisserand and Rodney Young are two leading figures in the world of aromatherapy, and this book is must-have for anyone who wants to expand the practice. More conservative than many sources, it provides in-depth safety information and encourages users to take care with essential oils.

Worwood, Valerie Ann. *The Complete Book of Essential Oils and Aromatherapy, Revised and Expanded: Over 800 Natural, Nontoxic, and Fragrant Recipes to Create Health, Beauty, and Safe Home and Work Environments.* Novato: New World Library, 2016.

More than just a simple guide to essential oils and aromatherapy, this book contains a treasure trove of information for dealing with a variety of issues. Valerie Ann Worwood has written a number of other books, all worth reading.

References

Abbas, Abul K., Andrew H. Lichtman, and Shiv Pillai. *Basic Immunology: Functions and Disorders of the Immune System.* 4th ed. Philadelphia: Saunders, 2012.

Appleton, Jeremy, ND. "Lavender Oil for Anxiety and Depression: Review of the Literature on the Safety and Efficacy of Lavender." *Natural Medicine Journal* 4, no. 2 (February 2012). Accessed August 18, 2017. www.naturalmedicinejournal.com/journal/2012-02/lavender-oil-anxiety-and-depression-0.

Boukhatem, Mohamed Nadjib, Mohamed Amine Ferhat, Abdelkrim Kameli, Fairouz Saidi, and Hadjer Tchoketch Kebir. "Lemongrass *(Cymbopogon citratus)* Essential Oil as a Potent Anti-Inflammatory and Antifungal Drug." *Libyan Journal of Medicine* 9 (2014). doi:10.3402/ljm.v9.25431.

Cooksley, Virginia Gennari. *Aromatherapy: A Lifetime Guide to Healing with Essential Oils.* Englewood Cliffs, NJ: Prentice Hall, 1996.

de Sousa, A. A., P. M. Soares, A. N. de Almeida, A. R. Maia, E. P. de Souza, and A. M. Assreuy. "Antispasmodic Effect of *Mentha Piperita* Essential Oil on Tracheal Smooth Muscle of Rats." *Journal of Ethnopharmacology* 130, no. 2 (July 20, 2010): 433–6. doi:10.1016/j.jep.2010.05.012. Epub May 19, 2010.

Edwards, Victoria H. *The Aromatherapy Companion: Medicinal Uses/Ayurvedic Healing/Body-Care Blends/Perfumes and Scents/Emotional Health and Well-Being.* North Adams: Storey Publishing, 1999.

Hay, I. C., M. Jamieson, and A. D. Ormerod. "Randomized Trial of Aromatherapy. Successful Treatment for Alopecia Areata." *Archives of Dermatology* 134, no. 11 (November 1998): 1349–52.

Juergens, U. R., M. Stöber, and H. Vetter. "The Anti-Inflammatory Activity of L-menthol Compared to Mint Oil in Human Monocytes in Vitro: A Novel Perspective for Its Therapeutic Use in Inflammatory Diseases." *European Journal of Medical Research* 3, no. 12 (December 16, 1998): 539–45.

Kianpour, M., A. Mansouri, T. Mehrabi, and G. Asghari. "Effect of Lavender Scent Inhalation on Prevention of Stress, Anxiety, and Depression in the Postpartum Period." *Iranian Journal of Nursing and Midwifery Research* 21, no. 2 (March–April 2016): 197–201. doi:10.4103/1735-9066.178248.

Keville, Kathi, and Mindy Green. *Aromatherapy: A Complete Guide to the Healing Art.* New York: Crossing Press, 2009.

Lawless, Julia. *The Illustrated Encyclopedia of Essential Oils.* New York City: HarperCollins, 1995.

Lillehei, Angela Smith, Linda L.Halcón, Kay Savik, and Reilly Reis. "Effect of Inhaled Lavender and Sleep Hygiene on Self-Reported Issues: A Randomized Controlled Trial." *Journal of Alternative and Complementary Medicine* 21, no. 7 (July 2015): 430–438. doi:10.1089/acm.2014.0327.

Lis-Balchin, Maria. *Aromatherapy Science: A Guide for Healthcare Professionals.* Grayslake: Pharmaceutical Press, 2006.

Pazyar, N., R. Yaghoobi, N. Bagherani, and A. Kazerouni. "A Review of Applications of Tea Tree Oil in Dermatology." *International Journal of Dermatology* 52, no. 7 (July 2013): 784–90. doi:10.1111/j.1365-4632.2012.05654.x. Epub September 24, 2012.

Pinto, Eugénia, Luís Vale-Silva, Carlos Cavaleiro, and Lígia Salgueiro. "Antifungal Activity of the Clove Essential Oil from *Syzygium aromaticum* on *Candida, Aspergillus*, and Dermatophyte Species." *Journal of Medical Microbiology* 58 (November 2009): 1454–1462. doi:10.1099/jmm.0.010538-0.

Price, Shirley. *Shirley Price's Aromatherapy Workbook*. London: Thorsons, 1993.

Shehad, Meg. "Rosewood, Lavender, and Clary Sage: What's the Connection?" Gritman Essential Oils. September 9, 2013. Accessed August 10, 2017. www.gritman.com/blog/rosewood-lavender-and-clary-sage-whats-the-connection/.

Tisserand Institute. "Dilution Guidelines for Essential Oils." 2015. Accessed August 26, 2017. http://tisserandinstitute.org/wp-content/uploads/2015/01/EO-dilution.pdf.

Tisserand, Robert, and Rodney Young. *Essential Oil Safety: A Guide for Health Care Professionals*. 2nd ed. Edinburgh: Churchill Livingstone, 2013.

Tisserand, Robert B. *The Art of Aromatherapy: The Healing and Beautifying Properties of the Essential Oils of Flowers and Herbs*. New York City: Simon & Schuster (Healing Arts Press), 1978.

U.S. Department of Health and Human Services: National Institutes of Health, National Center for Complementary and Integrative Health. "Peppermint Oil." Accessed August 13, 2017. nccih.nih.gov/health/peppermintoil.

Warad, Shivaraj B., Sahana S. Kolar, Veena Kalburgi, and Nagaraj B. Kalburgi. "Lemongrass Essential Oil Gel as a Local Drug Delivery Agent for the Treatment of Periodontitis." *Ancient Science of Life* 32, no. 4 (April 2013): 205–11. doi:10.4103/0257-7941.131973.

WebMD. "Frankincense." Accessed August 12, 2017. www.webmd.com /vitamins-supplements/ingredientmono-448-FRANKINCENSE.aspx ?activeIngredientId=448&activeIngredientName=FRANKINCENSE.

Worwood, Valerie Ann. *The Complete Book of Essential Oils and Aromatherapy, Revised and Expanded: Over 800 Natural, Nontoxic, and Fragrant Recipes to Create Health, Beauty, and Safe Home and Work Environments.* Novato: New World Library, 2016.

Index

248

Acknowledgments

To David, who cleans house, does dishes, and provides outstanding moral support while I'm busy writing, I am so very thankful. You have my heart.

To Clara Song Lee, with sincere gratitude for being a helpful, supportive editor. Also to the editing and design team for their efforts: It truly takes a village to create a book! My appreciation knows no bounds.

To Shannon, Kenya, Devon, Ben, and the rest of the wonderful staff at my favorite Barnes and Noble location, thank you for welcoming me into your café so often. Working in an active environment prevents cabin fever and the drinks are an enormous help.

Last but not least, a huge thanks and all my love to my parents, Tom and Lynn, who raised me to think critically and take risks, while accepting challenges.

About the Author

ANNE KENNEDY is an independent writer who enjoys covering a wide variety of topics, including natural health, simple living, sustainability, and gardening, across an array of markets. She has written several books on essential oils and herbal medicine, including *Aromatherapy for Natural Living* and *The Portable Essential Oils*.

Self-sufficiency; an active outdoor lifestyle; and a strong focus on the interconnectedness of body, mind, and spirit serve as her inspiration and her cornerstones for healthy living. Her lifelong study of herbs and plants began during her childhood in Montana's Bitterroot Valley, beginning with an interest in Native American herbal remedies. Her study of essential oils and aromatherapy was inspired by her initial exposure to lavender essential oil and her intrigue at just how effectively it remedies a variety of everyday issues.

Anne lives and works from her home on a small organic farm in the mountains of West Virginia. Her favorite essential oil is frankincense.

31901062470945

9 781939 754608